It Takes
You
to Tango

*Leverage the science of loneliness
to master the art of connection*

Amit Sood, MD

A three-step approach to tame your inner bully,
build self-worth, and nurture self-love.

Copyright © 2024 Amit Sood, MD

All rights reserved.

ISBN: 978-1-7347377-6-9

This publication is in copyright. No part of this book may be reproduced or transmitted in any form or by any means without the written permission of the author.

Disclaimer: The information in this book is not intended to substitute a physician's advice or medical care. Please consult your physician or other health care provider if you are experiencing any symptoms or have questions pertaining to the information contained in this book.

DANCE, AND THE WORLD
WILL *DANCE* WITH YOU

To all the world's pets, dogs in particular!

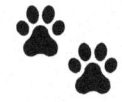

Contents

Introduction 9
Your Three Relationships 19
    1 Connect-In 20
    2 RUM 24
    3 Your Three Relationships 30
    4 D to C 35
    5 Your Best Friend 39
    6 North Star 42
    7 Hello Others 47
Step I Shed Self-Rejection 53
    8 Why Self-Rejection? 54
    9 Guilt (and Shame) 63
    10 Taming Your Guilt (and Shame) 70
Step II Build Self-Worth 80
    11 Knowing Self-Worth 81
    12 Why Did I Forget? 86
    13 Our Comparison Instinct 89
    14 Hurtful Comparisons 92
    15 Helpful Comparisons 95
Step III Nurture Self-Love 101
    16 Understanding Self-Love 102
    17 Say No To Life Limiters 109
Your "Self": A Model 115
    18 Self, An Introduction 116
    19 Build or Break? 120
    20 What Do You Think? 126
    21 Your Presence 131

22 Our Complex Psyche 135

Self-Compassion **142**

23 What Is Self-Compassion? 143

24 Common Barriers to Self-Compassion 151

25 Three Levels 158

26 Self-Trust 162

27 Imposter Phenomenon 166

28 Actionable Insights 175

29 Self-Compassion Practices 184

Self-Acceptance **196**

30 Eight Billion Sages 197

31 What Is Self-Acceptance? 203

32 Self-Acceptance: Why 208

33 Self-Acceptance: How (Insights) 212

34 Self-Acceptance: How (Practices) 217

Self-Forgiveness **227**

35 This You Know Already 228

36 The Five Steps 233

A Covenant With Self **239**

Epilogue **241**

Appendix A Loneliness Basics **244**

Appendix B How Loneliness Perpetuates Itself **247**

Appendix C Loneliness and Connection with Self **249**

Appendix D What Works? **252**

Notes **256**

Acknowledgements **287**

About The Author **288**

Introduction

> Pause for a moment and meet yourself, without the noise of your past regrets and others' judgments. You might like what you see. It might be the start of a lifelong friendship...with the self.

At the southern tip of Washington state, nestled between the Pacific Ocean on the west, Columbia River on the south, and Willapa Bay on the east, is the three-mile-wide Long Beach Peninsula. Once a prosperous salmon-fishing community, decades of overfishing have forced the region to rely on tourists who love to fly kites and drive along the thirty-mile-long hard sand beach hugging the ocean. I was fortunate to serve that community as a country doctor from 1997 to 2003.

It was love at first sight for me, both with the place and the people. Long Beach offered the perfect combination of a naturally picturesque landscape, simple, kind people, and the mighty Pacific singing a soft lullaby every night. The clinical practice was also rewarding with one caveat. Patients often brought homegrown cucumbers as their copay!

One day at the office, a hurried knock startled me while I was trying to decipher a patient's heart murmur during his annual physical.

I apologized to the patient and stepped out to discover a grinning Cindy, my conscientious and extraordinarily skilled nurse.

"You've got to see this, Dr. Sood. You have a surprise visitor." Cindy scurried me to the next room.

A middle-aged lady with an ear-to-ear smile sat on the chair, her hair in a neat bun and a small bunny in her lap.

"Is that Donna?" I was glad I remembered her name.

"That's me!" She got up with Coco (her bunny) tucked on her side and gently hugged me. Coco's wet nose rubbed against my sanitized hands.

"Your prescription worked like magic," Donna said, showing me a wrinkled piece of paper with a year-old script in my handwriting.

Patient: *Donna Davison*

Rx: *Get a pet ASAP x 1*

Refills authorized: *As needed (for life)*

Signed: Dr. Amit Sood, MD MS FACP
Date: xx / xx / 2001

Seeing that prescription rekindled all my memories.

I had started seeing Donna as a patient, a sixty-year-old retired teacher, about three years ago. During her visits, she mostly talked about her husband, who had lost his lungs to a lifetime of smoking, a carryover from the battlefields of Vietnam. Their only son lived somewhere in Southern California but seldom called.

Donna came every month for about a year to get a written script for her medicines, but mostly to talk about her husband. She insisted on in-person visits, but after about a year, she stopped coming.

A few weeks later, after reading her husband's obituary in the local newspaper, I called Donna but couldn't reach her. I sent her a condolence letter and then got busy keeping the practice afloat.

Several months later, Donna reappeared as a walk-in to get her ears checked. She didn't have any ear symptoms but wanted me to peek anyway. "Your ears are just fine," I said as I looked at her healthy tympanic membranes with my otoscope. She shrugged her shoulders, but without saying much, she left.

A week later, I saw her again with the same request. After her third "ear-visit" in three weeks, Cindy suggested, "Maybe she comes for the connection. Could she be feeling lonely?" That's when the lightbulb in my head, half snuffed from my pharmacotherapy-focused medical training, turned on.

I tried different ways to connect Donna with the community, but she wasn't interested in boasting about her Bingo wins or hearing World War II stories. Therapist appointments were out for six months since they prioritized seeing sad and anxious youth, of which there were plenty in my community with its median income hugging the poverty line.

With few options left, Donna and I reluctantly surrendered to an antidepressant. She liked the medicine, not because of its mood benefits, but because of a desirable GI side effect — it fixed her constipation!

Running out of ideas, on a whim one day, I wrote on my prescription pad, "Get a pet ASAP."

I'm glad she didn't take my non-formulary script to the pharmacy. Her insurance company would have denied the coverage. Instead, she drove to a rabbit rescue facility. She had long dreamed of having a bunny and feeding him home-grown carrots that her teeth could no longer chew.

A year out from that day, there was Donna, with an ear-to-ear smile I still remember twenty-three years later.

That was 2001 when I last met Donna, and the first time my mind opened to my patients' struggle with loneliness, a word unfamiliar to me as a recent immigrant from New Delhi, India.

From where I came, even if you wanted to feel alone you couldn't. The moment you stepped out of your home, you were surrounded by a sea of humanity and a myriad of other species. This could either be a feast for your eyes or sensory overload depending on your social appetite and tolerance for chaos.

Loneliness, from what I recall, was not mentioned even once in my twelve years of medical training, overseas and in the U.S. You couldn't become a tenured "Professor of Loneliness."

Nevertheless, learning from Donna's experience, I quickly adjusted my reference frame. I started looking for loneliness around me. To my surprise, hidden behind a thin veil, I found it everywhere: in teachers, physical therapists, hospital administrators, fishermen, farmers, students, and more.

Over the next few months, the repertoire of my non-pharmacologic prescriptions expanded: get a talking Furby; consider volunteering at the hospital; join a book club; host a community Thanksgiving dinner; take in an exchange student; go for a walk in the local mall.

My patients loved my non-drug prescriptions, seeing them as a nudge to bring more joy and connection to their lives. At my end, I was heeding Dr.

William Osler's admonition: "The person who takes medicine must recover twice, once from the disease and once from the medicine." I wanted my patients to need recovery only once.

As the years rolled by, however, my prescriptions lost their impact. "Perhaps they have lost novelty," I thought. "Or has my handwriting become illegible?" I had heard jokes about doctors' handwriting, which is often atrocious, compared to the bills which are all neatly typewritten. Little did I know that something deeper and more sinister was at play.

A newer, hardier form of loneliness was emerging with people feeling lonely in the company of each other. This modern loneliness wasn't related to an absence of social connections. It occurred from a combination of an inner disconnection and a lack of nurturing, uplifting, high-quality social contact. No wonder it couldn't be helped by simply increasing the number of people my patients met in a day. On the contrary, sometimes they felt lonelier in others' presence.

At first, it didn't quite make sense. But when I looked at the macro world, two changes were happening — Tech stocks (like Yahoo and Amazon) were soaring, and mental health was declining.

Globally, technology was accelerating the pace of change in people's lives. The world's most brilliant minds were busy innovating algorithms, so you click more ads, not spread compassion and forgiveness.

Further, by every measure, mental health was declining — teenage drug use, deaths by suicide, prevalence of mood disorders, use of antidepressants and anti-anxiety pills. The rapidity of change and the accompanying stress was systematically redesigning the human brain, unfortunately not in a salutary way.

The brain's higher cortical part, which helps you cultivate compassion, handle complexity, flexibly adapt to change, and exercise self-control, was getting weaker. Simultaneously, the lower limbic part, the one that hosts hostility, anger, and fear, was getting stronger. "Why would our brain allow itself to be maladaptively redesigned?" I wondered.

Fortunately, science had advanced enough to give me some answers. The concept of neuroplasticity, your brain's ability to change with experience, was now firmly entrenched in the scientific world.

Instead of mind over matter, scientists were figuring out how experience turns mind into matter. Here is how the neuroplasticity-generated positive feedback loop was creating a momentum problem in our brain.

Step 1: The brain engages in a particular practice (e.g., learning to play the piano).
Step 2: The brain circuits that host this practice become stronger.
Step 3: With more robust brain circuits, you become good at that practice and start enjoying it, eventually spending more time with it, both learning and practicing.

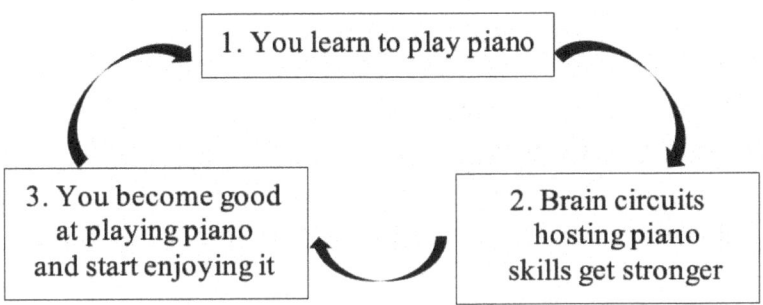

Do you see how neuroplasticity-based learning creates a valuable positive feedback loop that allows you to be simultaneously awesome and a work in progress?

However, what if that initial experience, instead of playing piano, was the fear of public speaking?

Neuroplasticity is a two-way process; it can be as easily harmful as it is helpful. For instance, re-evaluate the accompanying figure with "the fear of public speaking." The more you fear, the stronger the brain's fear network, which makes you fear even more. That is the basis of an anxiety-provoking moment becoming a panic attack.

The cumulative effect of uncertainty, ambiguity, and polarization in our world now compounds our brain's vulnerability. Further, the human brain is the engine that powers economic progress. A rise in GDP and brain overload are thus inseparable. As a result, our brains now must lift the equivalent of a hundred pounds of cognitive and emotional load all day long.

A few obvious sources of the load (not in order of importance) are:

- increasing social comparisons
- greater exposure to the world's (negative) news
- excessive screen time

- a greater potential to achieve extrinsic goals through capitalistic drive (money, fame, success) creating perpetual FOMO (Fear of Missing Out)
- accelerating pace causing a change overdose
- loss of trust in each other and institutions
- a mushrooming of conspiracy theories
- increasing income disparity
- a polarizing political environment
- increasing narcissism
- breaking down of stable relationships
- high expectations among youth
- lingering effects of childhood trauma
- global events (the pandemic, wars, economy, racial divide)

The modern brains carry many more open files than our hunter-gatherer ancestors. No wonder people have no dispensable attention or energy left to connect with others or themselves.

A combination of these changes has set us on a downward mental health spiral that shows no signs of letting up. A decline in mental health hurts all our relationships, including the most sacred and precious one — with ourselves.

Losing that final support, we are now amidst a mental health crisis, with the pandemic providing the tailwinds just at the wrong time.

We need to stop this downward spiral, which will entail a concerted and thoughtful effort that is broad in scope and enduring.

So, I was elated to see the diversity of brilliance at the March 2024 World Well-being Forum on loneliness at the London School of Economics and the World Happiness Summit (WOHASU), held at the Southbank's Queen Elizabeth Hall in London. I attended and presented a keynote at the event.[1]

In the august presence of some of the who's who of the loneliness and well-being sciences — Professor Lord Richard Layard, Tracey Crouch (World's First Minister for Loneliness), U.S. Surgeon General Dr. Vivek Murthy, Professor Arthur Brooks, and many others — I learned and shared the latest in well-being and loneliness insights. Each speaker offered ideas that together could be summarized in the following four key points:

- The world is simultaneously getting more populous and lonelier

- A perceived lack of connections is as damaging to physical health as smoking cigarettes and is worse than a sedentary lifestyle
- Poor mental health and disconnection feed into each other
- Building relationships is a global public health priority but we are presently unsure how best to bring us all together

With over 15,000 papers on the topic, the research community has done a fantastic job of highlighting the importance of loneliness. We have demonstrated the impact of disconnection on neural circuitry, inflammatory gene expression, and daily behaviors. In hundreds of studies, we have shown how a sense of isolation hurts our mental health and workplace engagement, increases our risk for chronic diseases, and decreases our health and life span. We have also begun implementing all this knowledge to improve our connections — by reimagining our built spaces, rewriting government policies, and revamping employment benefits. Yet, despite all our good intentions, rigorous science, and political will, more teenagers and adults feel lonely today than ever before.

Why this disconnect? Importantly, what if our current efforts aren't addressing the core issues at play?

As I reviewed the research, a few additional questions troubled me. Why do professionals like flight attendants and healthcare providers who might meet hundreds of people daily still feel lonely? How does the brain's innate response to loneliness perpetuate disconnection? How does our relationship with ourselves influence our relationship with others? How do we meaningfully connect with others if we are disconnected from ourselves?

In this book, I answer some of these questions and, in the process, start creating a path out of this quagmire. I share that <u>the most important relationship to curb your loneliness is your connection with yourself</u>.

Our low self-worth, mental health concerns, poor self-care, and deficits in kindness all relate to an inner loneliness that has been around for a long time but has recently taken the center stage.

<u>Inner loneliness is lacking a positive nurturing connection with oneself</u>. It originates in negative self-judgments that lead to self-rejection and disconnection. Increasing the "dose" of outer connections does very little to improve inner loneliness.

All our lives, we look out for someone to support, inspire, and cherish us, not realizing that we are looking for ourselves. Thus, the first step to a meaningful loneliness solution is to overcome self-rejection and disconnection, by developing a kinder, more accepting, compassionate, and forgiving disposition toward oneself.

But that's not what I entertained until a few years ago. My former self believed that self-compassion was for the weak; self-forgiveness was for those unwilling to take responsibility. Self-love seemed perfectly appropriate to decorate the cover of well-being magazines we skim at hairdressing salons, but otherwise sounded hollow.

However, as a person of science, when I looked at the data, I found two impressive lines of evidence that provided a call to action:

1. Study after study showed how much we struggle with low self-worth and lack of self-compassion.
2. Research showed the striking benefits of enhancing self-compassion, self-acceptance, and self-forgiveness, not just for our mental health but for many physical, social, and work-related outcomes.

The final factor for me was when I sat down with two groups of people separately to understand their present struggles: middle schoolers and a cohort of resilience and well-being coaches.

I asked the middle schoolers to write down their present emotional struggles on Post-it notes and place them on the table. The data was striking. These giggly, happy-looking, easy-going kids suffered inside, mostly because of low self-worth. Despite a future filled with hope and possibilities, their present was riddled with feelings of despair.

With the resilience and well-being coaches, I asked two questions:

- What are your most pressing current emotional struggles?
- What would you tell your middle-schooler self if you were their counselor?

Again, the response was the same. Coaches' most significant emotional struggles related to low self-worth, feeling like an imposter, a lack of self-love, and loneliness. The most common words they wanted to say to their middle schooler self were, "You are enough."

"No matter our generation, age, or intellectual awareness, we all could benefit from a refresher in self-kindness," I concluded.

But why should masters of well-being — psychologists, wellness coaches, resilience experts — feel lonely and unworthy? Every single day, they help dozens of people overcome negative emotions. They certainly know how to support themselves emotionally and have no reason to feel unworthy given such a positive meaning to their work.

Interestingly, when I examined my innermost feelings, I found I was no better than many of my student resilience trainers. I felt as worthy as my most recent evaluation.

I wanted to exit this vulnerability but wasn't sure how. I was too afraid to let go of my perfectionism. I mistakenly felt that the best way to stay in the race was to keep flogging a tired horse (me).

From that personal need and the desire to help others, this book has emerged. It offers science, stories, and skills to help you move from an inner disconnection to an inner embrace of your "self." It is a reminder that your love for yourself seeds your love for others and their love for you. It is a covenant that helps you practice the simple principle that your relationship with yourself is the bedrock for all your other relationships. It offers you a conviction that self-compassion is a marker of your strength, not weakness, and self-trust is a sign of humility, not hubris.

The journey we will undertake will take you from shedding self-rejection to building self-worth and nurturing self-love, from inner loneliness to inner nurturing and connection.

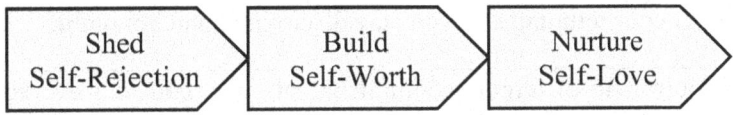

As we embark on our ride together, remember that the journey is often the destination, while what we define as a destination is another milestone.

You and I might experience one or more of the following welcome changes on our path.

Despite:

your previous mistakes or failures, you stay respectful of self.
things not going your way, you remain hopeful.
facing tough times, you find reasons for gratitude.
uncertainty of the results, you give your best.
a slow progress, you stay patient.
what others think of your looks, you feel beautiful, inside and outside.
others' many rejections, you continue loving yourself.
your several successes, you stay humble.
seeing others doing wrong, you do what's proper and ethical.
many fears in your mind, you stay courageous.
seeing others seek short-term success, you focus on your long-term purpose.
many pulls to your temptations, you stay disciplined and honorable.
meeting people with different accomplishments, you consider everyone equal.
the world mired in war, hatred, and revenge, you choose peace, love, and forgiveness.

I pray our time together empowers you, so you say *adieu* to self-doubt and self-judgment, always wake up in your nurturing company, and live each day inspired, full of hope, courage, and joy.

Let's turn the relationship clock back in our favor. Let's fall in love again, with ourselves!

Your Three Relationships

1
Connect-In

> Smile with your eyes and say hello. There is a one in two chance that the person in front of you feels vulnerable and lonely.

We seek happiness, health, respect, peace, purpose, and love. Many also crave dark chocolate!

From our very first wanderings on the planet, one common conduit has aided all human seeking — meaningful relationships (Figure 1). We are a social species for many good reasons.

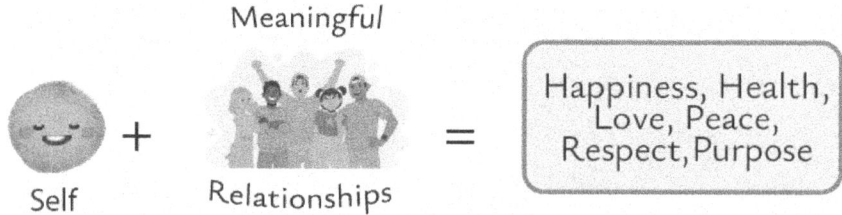

Figure 1. Meaningful relationships serve as a conduit to a good life

Unfortunately, of late, out of ignorance, ambition, and, in some instances, greed, we have started building a world where deep, nurturing relationships have gone backstage, replaced by superficial interactions.

At work, many of us spend 50 or more hours a week in a cubicle, meeting with people from across the world through two-dimensional rectangles. At home, slightly different screens absorb our evenings. Warm handshakes have become less common; ten-second hugs are rare.

This sudden change, an unintended consequence of industrialization, social mobility, and technological advancement, has upended every dimension of our lives. Our hard-earned meteoric rise in GDP in the last 50 years hasn't translated into any consequential gains in happiness. Our increase in lifespan has plateaued, with the last twenty percent of our life now spent struggling with a significant chronic illness. Trust is at or near an all-time low. Death by suicide is at or near an all-time high. Most of us lack a clear purpose for our lives. Every continent in the world is mired in conflicts. We can and must do better.

Healthcare professionals, researchers, entrepreneurs, and others have taken notice, developing myriad solutions to help rebuild our relationships. However, with few exceptions, our efforts to connect so far have produced unimpressive results.

While examining the underlying reasons for our failure and in search of new solutions, I discovered an intriguing set of research findings:

- Studies showed that higher amount of socializing may not protect people from lonely feelings.[1]
- People's loneliness was directly proportional to their number of meetings (the more meetings, the lonelier the workers felt).[2]
- Time together with others without a meaningful connection worsened people's loneliness.[3]
- Physicians felt similar or greater loneliness than people with visual or hearing impairment.[4-5]
- Multiple reviews of dozens of studies showed that helping people by providing more social support or social skills training only marginally improved loneliness.[6]

Intrigued by the data that showed the paradoxical effect of trying to increase connections on loneliness, I explored another line of research — the impact of connection with oneself on loneliness. Several studies showed that one of the strongest predictors of loneliness is a lack of a nurturing relationship with oneself. Thus, in dozens of studies, each of the following personal challenges predisposed to loneliness:

- Guilt and shame [7-10]
- Low self-worth [11-15]
- Lack of self-compassion [16-22]
- Lack of self-acceptance [23-25]
- Presence of psychiatric disorders (that predispose to all of the above) [26]
- Low emotional intelligence [27]

(Please see Appendix A and B for more details)

The above findings gave me three conclusions:

1. People with too many interactions but too few high-quality connections feel lonely.
2. The underlying cause of a broken relationship with others commonly is a fractured relationship with oneself, an inner loneliness that comes from self-rejection and lack of self-worth and self-love.
3. Improving relationship with oneself (through nurturing self-worth, self-trust, self-compassion, self-acceptance, and self-forgiveness) is an essential first step to improving relationships with others.

Our disconnect with ourselves, powered by upward comparisons, imposter phenomenon, toxic guilt, and lack of self-compassion, has been decades in the making. Let's see if, like me, you also got caught in this trap by carefully considering which of the following applies to you.

1. You are comfortable showing compassion to others but aren't good at being kind to yourself.
2. Sometimes, looking at others' social media accounts makes you feel small and unsuccessful.
3. You occasionally feel guilty even with little or no personal fault.
4. Despite working hard and succeeding in many ways, you feel like an imposter, thinking that one-day others might label you a fake.

If you answered yes to any of the above, let's redraw Figure 1 to emphasize the importance of a healthy inner connection (Figure 2).

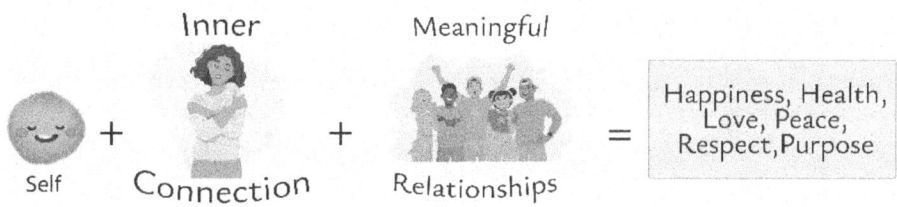

Figure 2. A healthy inner connection is the first step to a good life

Friend, your every worthwhile pursuit depends on a healthy inner connection that is brimming with self-worth and self-love. Until very recently, I was also caught in the swirl of self-rejection, living an imbalanced life. Let me start with excerpts from my story that I shared while trying to help one of my colleagues.

2
RUM

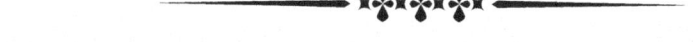

> You often judge yourself the most when you deserve the greatest compassion. Choose to be kind to yourself on those days.

Boyd grew up in Northern Minnesota with Lake Superior in his backyard. Belonging to a fishing family, he dreamed of earning enough money to buy a yacht, move to the Caribbean, and spend the rest of his life on the ocean. But a broken humerus from a fall changed his life's trajectory. In the hospital, he fell again, this time falling in love with a nurse and her chosen profession. He diverted his yacht money to medical school education and followed it with Emergency Medicine training.

When I met him, he was Dr. Boyd German, eighteen years into his career as an ER doctor. He had an excellent reputation for his clinical skills but was now facing disciplinary action. He had yelled at two of his patients because they didn't fill his prescription. Another day, a student recorded him threatening to punch an intern because of her "incompetence."

"I am already very resilient," he said with a stiff upper lip as he eased into the chair directly across me.

"Then why are you wasting my time? With that attitude, you're sure to lose your job." I would have said a decade ago. But now I knew that an expression other than love is a call for help.

"Sure, I get it. I'm here to listen and learn, more than suggest anything," I said.

"Are you part of admin? Is our conversation being recorded?" He looked around and surveyed the room.

"Neither. I am here to help, one colleague to another, because I was in your place a few years ago. Well, not exactly, but still not too different."

He seemed to like that.

Dr. German shuffled in his chair, then his eyes brightened. "Why not tell me your story."

"Sure," I said, unsure if he was really interested or just wanted to fill the time.

"I am married, have two daughters, and a dog. Most of my work is in the well-being and resilience space. But that's not how I started. As an internist, I practiced as a community doctor for several years. Life was going smoothly until a patient mishap became a two-year nightmare." Dr. German looked engaged.

"Long story short, I got an attorney's Dear Dr. Sood letter. Suddenly, from being respected and on top of my game, I felt like an outcast. It took two years to resolve, and by the time it was all clear, I knew who I could and couldn't trust. I was emotionally exhausted."

"What was the case? You don't have to share if it is confidential." I liked him asking questions but wanted to keep some boundaries. I knew he would respect me for that.

"It is somewhat confidential; I apologize," I responded. "Those two years, I felt very alone. But that was not the end of it. Before the dust settled, I experienced one after the other health crises in my family that culminated in a visit to the ER with my heart rate pushing 150."

"I am sorry to hear that."

"At some point along that journey, I realized that I need to take charge of my well-being. Nobody else would do that for me. I was running ten different research studies on top of a full clinical practice, being a good husband, dad, and son, and maintaining a perfect yard. I could have still managed it all if I was not a perfectionist go-getter."

"So, what did you do?"

"I'll share that in a moment. First, would you be okay sharing a bit about you?"

Dr. German nodded, cleared his throat, leaned back in his chair, and spoke. "Your story sounds like mine, in a way. I kid that I have five supervisors: my wife, my unit chief, my nurse, my patients, and my teenager. Every day, either one of them is unhappy with me, or I am with them. I can't recall a day when I didn't feel annoyed at someone's incompetence.

I don't feel good about myself. Sometimes, I think I should go back to my fishing days. Between balancing my work, research, education, and being a dad, husband, and son, I no longer know who I am. I am burnt out, man. I need to do something, but I don't know what."

He paused to collect his breath and stared into space. "My patients aren't the easiest either. Half of my community has no medical insurance. Their care starts and ends in the ER. That's not how it's supposed to be."

I nodded and looked away, giving him a little extra space.

After ten more minutes of conversation, I asked, "When was the last time you felt completely relaxed when you could shut off your phone and pager?"

He paused long and hard and said, "Like four years ago."

"What were you doing at that time?"

"I was under sedation, getting my colonoscopy."

We both broke into hilarious laughter. We needed that.

Sensing Dr. German was now ready to receive some suggestions, I started sharing self-management ideas. "Coming back to your question, what did I do to self-manage? I embraced the idea of being "good enough." I realized I could be perfect or awesome, not both. I chose to be awesome. I started sleeping more, took out time for workout, and prioritized my emotional well-being. I invested more time in my relationships, with others and most importantly, with myself. I became kinder to myself."

I paused, took a deep breath, and waited for Dr. German to respond. Seeing him interested and reflective, I shared more specific insights and skills.

"I deepened my neuroscience learning to understand my vulnerabilities. I realized that, like most others, I was spending up to 80 percent of my day with a wandering attention where my thoughts were generating neutral or negative feelings. I was amazed to learn that our brain tires after 90 minutes of sustained effort. Our brain isn't designed to log ten hours of work without rest. Just as your windshield collects dead bugs after driving 100 miles, your brain collects dead neurotransmitters after an hour or two, which interfere with its efficiency. Much of brain fatigue, however, is silent because your brain doesn't have any pain receptors for itself."

"Really! Tell that to my supervisor! How do you fix that? You have my ears for sure."

I decided to provide more background, sharing the gist of the insights and practices I use daily.[1]

"A few years ago, I researched an important question: what is our brain's core hunger beyond oxygen and glucose? I found three things. The first one is rest. Rest isn't figuring out your insurance coverage during your ten-minute break. A truly restorative rest happens when you let go of planning and problem-solving. The key is to let your adrenaline settle by not thinking about concerns and regrets and giving yourself freedom from addressing the 150 open files in your head."

"I get it. But I can't work for an hour and then rest for 30 minutes."

"Precisely! That's where the other two nutrients come in handy. The second one is uplifting emotions."

"Like what?"

"Anything that engages your brain's reward network — music, nature walks, deep breathing, meditation, reading a good book, listening to a devotional song, prayer, an uplifting phone call, watching family photos, reading grateful notes from your patients, or something else. The more active your engagement, the greater the benefit."

"Got it. What's the third hunger?"

"Motivation. Reminding yourself, why am I doing what I am doing? Once a brain has its why it doesn't need any other reward to fully engage with life."

"So, Rest, Uplifting emotions, and Motivation." I was impressed with Dr. German's focus and memory.

"Yes, and the acronym is RUM! I invite people to sip some RUM every hour or two."

"That's funny!" Dr. German laughed out loud. "I won't forget RUM! How do I bring more RUM into my life?"

"I suggest five ideas that are part of my daily routine now.[1] Let me summarize them and then I'm happy to go into details."

"Sure."

"First, right after I wake up, before I step on the carpet, I think about a few good people in my life and express my silent gratitude to them. I call this the morning gratitude practice. You can do it yourself or with the help of a YouTube video.[2]

"What if my head isn't clear or I have to rush to the bathroom?"

"Of course you can choose the specific time. I once woke up with my younger daughter's heel on my nose! Not the time to practice gratitude!

Second, at about 10 a.m., I take a short, "curious moments walk" around my office, noticing at least one interesting detail in the outside world. This practice gives a break to my brain's wandering attention.

Third, throughout the day, when I meet people, knowing that every person is special and has struggles, I send them a silent good wish instead of judging them."

"Doesn't it feel awkward to tell people, I wish you well?"

"Great question! The practice is silent. You don't say it. The goal is to silently connect with others and minimize the spot negative judgments you might make about them. Let's say you wish someone well, in addition to sending them a good wish, who is really benefited?"

"Me?"

"Precisely. Wishing others well is wishing yourself well. It doesn't take any time but helps you pull positive energy out of thin air. You can even take a short walk with the goal of sending a silent good wish to everyone you see. It is tremendously refreshing."

"I'll have to feel it to believe."

"Sure. Shall I share the fourth practice?" ER docs like to move fast!

"Sure."

"Meet your family at the end of the day as if you haven't seen them for a month — with good, warm energy. Try to notice your loved one's eye color when you meet them. Also, for the first two minutes, choose not to improve anybody. I call it the two-minute rule."

"You got me there. I'm always improving others." Dr. German and I both laughed.

"Yes, I did that too. But I realized that trying to improve others doesn't work and they start associating you with feeling bad about themselves. Also, storing old grudges isn't a good use of your brain's premium real estate. Instead, when you help them feel worthy, they will start seeking and liking you. In fact, you can use this practice with your interns, patients, and others. Start at home and gradually expand to work." I could see Dr. German connecting the dots.

"Finally, before sleeping at night, I send good energy to someone I met during the day who I felt was struggling. You can pray for them or just send them a positive healing intention, whatever you prefer.

In other words, start your day with gratitude and end with compassion. Remember that because of the way the human brain operates, the pursuit of compassion will make you happier than the pursuit of happiness."

"I like the simplicity and brevity, but I bet it must be very powerful. I'll try at least a couple of ideas," Dr. German said. I was happy to earn his trust.

I wrote all the practices on a paper and invited Dr. German to mark one or two that made the most sense to him. He picked the morning gratitude and the two-minute rule (meeting family for the first two minutes as if he hadn't seen them for a month with no desire to improve them). I took him through the morning gratitude practice as a three-minute meditation and shared more details about the two-minute rule.

We planned a four-week follow-up to continue working on better managing emotions. Just as he was leaving, he turned around and asked, "What do you do with all those worries?"

"We will talk about them in the next visit. For now, consider practicing the Scheduled Worry Time. To put it simply, schedule your worries once or twice a day when you give them your full attention. If they ping your brain at other times, tell yourself I have set aside time for this again tomorrow."

"Will that cut my worries, just like that?"

"Not always, but early research is promising. I implemented scheduling my worries when I realized that I was worrying that I wasn't worrying! I also now try to remember that while my worries fight the shadows, it is my courage that fights the monster. I carefully choose my soldier."

"One more question. Was I wrong in thinking I was resilient?"

"No, you weren't. But today, people from every walk of life are struggling. It is because since childhood, while we learn skills to be effective and efficient at work, we get minimal training in how to manage our emotions and connection with ourselves. Most people do not fail because they forget the basics of their job. They struggle with emotions, connections, and self-worth. That's why I focus on these aspects in my approach to resilience."

"That makes sense. Also, teaching people about their brain fatigue and mind wandering removes some stigma."

"Precisely. A lot of the stigma exists because our brain is remarkably good at believing in those who don't believe in us. Tell me, who loves you unconditionally? Someone in whose presence you never have to pretend."

"Promise you won't tell this to my wife." Dr. Boyd had a twinkle in his eyes.

"I promise."

"My dog, Bruno!" We both smiled.

"Until we meet next, try to look at yourself with Mr. Bruno's eyes. You are who your pet thinks you are."

3
Your Three Relationships

> All relationships at work and home can improve once you remember this simple rule — each person you meet is special and struggling.

Dogs. They love you more than they love themselves. I have reveled in their authentic unconditional love since my teenage years. My Goldendoodle, Simba, is absolutely untainted and one hundred percent authentic. He gets so excited when I come home that he occasionally wets the floor while listening to my car pulling in! Not even Richa (my lovely wife), who loves a nice-smelling living room, minds the occasional tropical islands he creates. "They are a tapestry of love," she says.

Like our pets, young children are also authentic if we adults do not douse their authenticity. One of my primary parental responsibilities is to help my girls (Gauri and Sia) stay true to themselves as they discover their world. That entails an egalitarian home environment, giving them a strong say in how Richa and I are present in their company.

Before we get too deep into this book, I want to share an important practice I have found very helpful. Its basis is the concept of autonomy threat.[1] Children and adults want to feel capable and in control. When they feel babied or overly controlled, they feel threatened and, in reaction, stop cooperating. So, I try to let them carry the baton as long as they can. Here is how this specific practice works.

Every quarter, I request Gauri and Sia to provide me with a "360-degree feedback" on my performance as a dad. I have received wonderfully humbling comments over the years. "Floss more often, dad." "Let mom teach you how to load the dishwasher." "The more you ask me about my crush, the less I want to talk about it." "Your accent isn't bad, but I suggest you stop saying echo as eeecho." Ouch!

I take their feedback as a message that they care about me. Taking their feedback and acting on it helps me dismantle their autonomy threat. Thus, every change I make based on their feedback gives me a pass to offer them a little suggestion and be taken seriously — a true win-win.

I worry, however, that the world is losing its authenticity, and thus, its innocence. Given the mushrooming of alternative facts, fake AI-created content, productivity pressures in academics that promote dishonesty, and more, I don't know who or what to trust anymore. Falsehood peddling with the resulting loss of trust has increased polarization and conflicts. Yet, looking at history, I stay hopeful, given humanity's collective ability to ensure that truth eventually prevails.

The truth matters. An unpleasant truth serves you better than a pleasant lie. However, everyone's truth is slightly different. A book writes its truth afresh every time a new person reads it since they interpret it with their veritas. So, as you and I co-author this book, let's promise to stay faithful to each other. I'll share what I have learned and experienced without bias or judgment. Further, I'll only share practices I have tried or am willing to embrace. I invite you to evaluate all my words with your core values. Throw away anything that doesn't make sense and embrace what does.

Let me start by challenging your math ability and introducing you to an "alternative" math equation that my first teacher, my mother, taught me.

One plus one equals eleven

What is one plus one in relationships?" My eighty-nine-year-old mother, Shashi, asked me at the dinner table. We were talking about the value of connections for overcoming life's struggles. Despite her fading memory, Shashi's retired middle school teacher self rejoices in flooring me with trick questions that have an obvious answer which is never the correct one.

"It is two, Mom," I gave the mathematically correct answer. I knew what was coming.

"No, it is eleven!" she said with her chin up, her head bobbing in a meaningful nod.

"How so?" I asked, amused.

She kept two forks side by side and looked at me with a triumphant smile, "Do you see eleven? When two people join forces, their power grows tenfold."

"What about one plus one plus one?" I playfully challenged her.

Another fork appeared. "It becomes one hundred and eleven!"

By now, thousands of research studies have proven my mother's wisdom. Relationships impact every single health measure, from molecules to mind to mortality.[2-5] Relationships, however, were the last thing on my mind as I relocated to the United States in the summer of 1995.

Relocating

I moved to the U.S. in June 1995, hoping to learn from the best in the world. I had a once-in-a-lifetime opportunity to work alongside researchers and clinicians who had authored many of my medical textbooks. As my airplane landed at the JFK airport, I was both excited and worried. I was excited to meet the wise professors but worried about how we would discern each other's accents.

At that time, I had a negative bank balance. New York also seemed like a different planet. The only thing common between New York and New Delhi was the word New. Otherwise, they were poles apart. For example, the central area of the city is called a *bazaar* in New Delhi, not downtown. To me, going downtown meant going downstairs! Machines swallowing dollars and giving nothing back in return and bottled water costing more than a can of soda made no sense. I was also unaware of the familiar East Coast prayer, "God give me patience, but please hurry up!"

The change in weather confused my hypothalamus. I had arrived from a sweltering 110 degrees in New Delhi, where my concrete dwelling would never cool up, not even at night. Most afternoons, you could make an omelet by cracking an egg on the street. New York City's 50 degrees at night was foreign to my frame. On top of that was the confusing technology. American electrical switches didn't follow the British design, which was the standard I had learned. Further, working at 40 percent of its capacity, my jet-lagged brain made everything less 'figureoutable.'

Not knowing how to operate the heating, I spent my first night in a cold basement apartment with a handkerchief of a blanket. When I covered my chest, everything below my knees froze. I switched around, only to experience my fingers turning tingly blue. The fetal position gave me a few good snores, but an urge to stretch my legs brought me back to square one.

Two decades out, balancing my life felt the same. A wisp of a hiatus from figuring out my children's activities was interrupted by the dentist's voicemail. I had missed a cleaning visit. The moment I heaved a sigh of relief on clearing credit card bills, from the corner of my eyes I spied the word "Delinquent" inscribed in bold red on an official-looking paper. It was a utility disconnect notice. My checking account was likely in overdraft, so the bank stopped paying the bills. It's a good thing the expression work-life balance is out of fashion. I was never a fan.

So, here was my unsurprising conclusion: my life was out of balance. I wasn't scheduling my priorities; I was prioritizing what landed on my schedule. Other than sleep, I didn't have any assigned downtime. Work and responsibilities had taken over my hours, like the salt in an over-salted soup.

One day several winters ago (that's how we measure time in Minnesota), while looking for solutions, I donned my resilience and well-being "expert" hat and closely examined my life — specifically my relationships.

My relationships

After much thinking, I realized that three core relationships helped me feel fulfilled and captured most of my daily interactions. They were with:

1. Myself
2. Others
3. Purpose

Myself: How was I relating with me? Was I treating myself with compassion, acceptance, love, and forgiveness, or self-judgment and rejection?

Others: Others included my loved ones, friends, neighbors, colleagues, clients, and the larger world. Was I treating others with respect, care, and love, or anger, envy, and disregard?

Purpose: Fortunately, I have had a clear purpose guiding my life for almost two decades — *to help build a kinder, happier, and more hopeful world for our planet's children.* But it takes a sustained disciplined effort to convert purpose into action and accomplishment. Were my daily activities aligned with my purpose or was I distracted, disengaged, and divergent?

With this clarity of questions, I set out to assess how I was doing in these three relationships.

4
D to C

> Birds with asymmetric feathers are the only ones that can fly. Assume that your life's present asymmetries may be pushing you to greater heights.

Here is my honest, down-to-earth assessment based on my overall performance over the years.

With myself: I frequently judged my intentions and performance, felt like an imposter, and held myself to unachievable standards. I gravitated to negative self-talk and seldom paused to smell the roses. I rarely enjoyed my company and often resorted to distracting activities so I could escape my presence.
My grade: D

With others: I was hurried, impatient, and judgmental. I interacted with many but had few, if any, authentic connections, striving instead to network only with the "important" people who could benefit me. I wasn't paranoid but often assumed negative intent, feeling judged in others' presence. Most of my connections weren't mutually uplifting or nurturing.
My grade: C

With my life's purpose: Despite being innately altruistic, I was caught in predominantly hedonic pursuits. In most engagements, I looked for personal gains. I worried others would construe my generosity as my naïveté.
My grade: C

You can see why I felt out of balance. A close-knit family, many good people in one's life, and a respected profession do not always translate into a feeling of belonging. I knew that now. I felt alone and fake for teaching some of the same skills I was lacking.

I resolved to mend my life by working on my three relationships. The obvious starting point was my relationship with others. Little did I know that I was heading straight into the swirls of a neural trap.

Loneliness trap

Three words capture the definition of loneliness: Unmet connection needs. Loneliness is of two types: short-term and long-term (or chronic). Short-term loneliness, which you might experience on a weekend, prompts a desire to connect. You reach out to someone that leads to a dinner date or watching a game together. You are back to life's scenic highway.

The chronic loneliness (one that lasts for months or years), however, evokes a different response that can lay a trap.[1] Chronically lonely people start seeing social connections as a source of rejection. Their mental health worsens; they stop trusting others. They also do not seek help because they fear being stigmatized.[2-3] Because of this social sensitivity, they avoid connecting, which leads to persistent disconnection and thus ongoing loneliness. Figure 3 shows how this trap operates. (Please see Appendix C for a summary of research.)

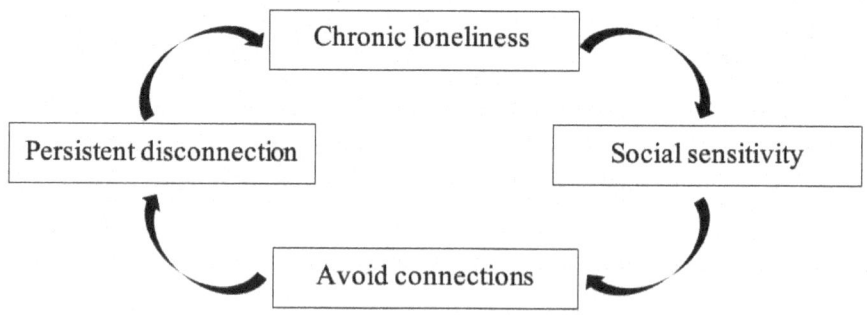

Figure 3. The feedback loop that creates loneliness trap

The loneliness trap nicely explains why trying to increase connections only modestly helps a chronically lonely person.

At my end, the more I tried to escape the loneliness trap, the stronger it pulled me. Two immediate challenges blocked my progress:

1. I couldn't loosen up enough to make meaningful connections (my non-trusting, fearful brain stuck in the loneliness trap wasn't ready to be vulnerable).
2. Others weren't available.

Let me elaborate on the second point because of its daily relevance. Many of us are busy handling multiple open files in our heads. The result is a state of constant distraction. Since we master what we practice for decades (neuroplasticity), our brains now struggle with giving anyone our sustained attention.

Also, because of widespread mental fatigue (resulting from an unrested brain), we do not have as much pep as we did a decade ago. A recent article correctly elaborated on the phenomenon of languishing, which affects almost two out of three people today.[4]

Please don't take it the wrong way. I'm not blaming anyone; blaming helps no one and depletes willpower. I very likely treat others the same. My goal is to get to the bottom of the problem so I can help others and myself. Having studied resilience and neuroscience for two decades, I think the problem relates to clogging. Let me explain.

Mental clog

Our brain's short-term memory that holds information for processing (its computer equivalent being the RAM) has a finite capacity. It is clogged these days with too many open files.[5-6] These files crowd our attention even when we aren't actively processing them. You may have felt its effect, when after a full day of work, you can't shut your mind off in the evening, even though you are with family and want to be fully present.

In personal relationships, people also struggle with the classic demand-withdrawal complex — the more you want others' attention, the more they withdraw, which makes you want more, making them withdraw even more.

My failure to raise my relationship grade with others had an additional unanticipated effect. My other two grades (my relationship with myself and with my purpose) started inching toward an F.

That's when I thought about changing the sequence. How about connecting with myself first, then moving to purpose and relationships? I liked this idea because to connect with myself, I needed just me to move forward. It entailed going inward and changing my perceptions instead of expecting the outside world to change.

But I wasn't sure. Would it lead to greater loneliness and a feeling of disconnection? Would I become too self-absorbed? I didn't know the answer but was up for the challenge — with one caveat. I didn't want to become a Minnesotan hermit. I had not traveled all the way from the land of the Himalayas to now Uber Eats my meals in the Midwest cornfields.

Thankfully, my mind didn't let that happen. It had something to do with donuts.

Unappetizing donuts?

A few years ago, in the middle of a respiratory infection, I transiently lost my taste sensation. The infection also caused a sustained bitter taste in my mouth. Nothing tasted good then, even donuts. That got me thinking about taste perception — it has as much to do with the state of my mouth as it does with the food. As a student of the mind, I wondered if that's how my other life experiences also play out.

If my mind is bitter, I fail to experience the love flowing from the world. Just as the flavor of every morsel depends on my taste buds, similarly, my mind colors everything I see and hear. As a result, I do not experience the world as it is. I experience it as my mind shows it to me.

As they say, just wear good shoes instead of removing all the rocks from the earth. Similarly, you can't change every relationship, but you can work on the mind that perceives them.

Working on your mind is essential because no amount of love coming from the world would matter unless you have a healthy relationship with yourself — the topic of our next conversation.

5

Your Best Friend

> If a few people have firmly decided to dislike you, trying to change their opinion will be a waste of time. Focus on the rest eight billion.

"Let's do a little practice now." I was presenting a mainstage keynote on "The connection cure" at the 2024 annual American Psychological Association (APA) meeting in Seattle, WA.

"Please speak your best friend's name. Loud as you can!"

The auditorium got boisterous. It took a little effort before I could reestablish peace. People like to talk!

"Now, please take out your smartphone and turn on the camera. Flip the camera and smile into it." I paused so everyone could join in. "The person you are seeing on the screen is your best friend. It's YOU!"

I heard a roar, like a 737 taking off. People got it and hopefully will not forget this important lesson. *You are your best friend.* Just as your heart serves itself before nourishing the body, you must take care of yourself first to continue serving the world.

If that's the truth, then why don't we treat ourselves with the same gentleness and care with which we treat our friends, loved ones, clients, and others? Why does it take zero effort to negatively judge the self while worthiness feels like a tall mountain to climb?

Scientists offer many reasons.
- We know our inner thoughts and find it easy to disapprove of them

- We fear that by accepting the self we will give ourselves a free pass
- We have a negativity bias that forces us to focus on our imperfections
- We feel the negative is more actionable, so focusing on our shortcomings is a good way to overcome them
- We give no pushback when self-critical, but others don't receive critiques that easily

Because of the above reasons, negative self-judgment is an effortless default for us. I do have an additional neuroscience-based theory.

Who is judging whom?

When you judge yourself, your higher cortical brain (the prefrontal cortex) engages and does the judging. And who does it evaluate? It looks down (literally) at your lower limbic brain (the amygdala), which is the seat of negative emotions. It is like a sage judging an alligator for its values. The alligator is bound to come short.

The prefrontal cortex also scans your hippocampus and other memory areas for stored recollections. In that autobiography are some dark pages — of the prank you played on your substitute teacher, the lie you told to avoid the parking ticket, the day you got drunk and... I'll spare the details!

That's not all. Social media feeds, plentiful in our world now, are phenomenally effective at generating toxic comparisons. When we compare our chapter three to someone's chapter thirty-four, which we often do, we are bound to come short. Every such comparison damages a few neurons in the brain's reward areas. Further, the resulting imposter feelings and envy hurt their owners' endocrine and cardiovascular systems.

Envy feels stifled if it must stay silent. It likes to show its fangs in the form of harsh words and actions. Behind the anonymity of user IDs, people feel safe and comfortable unleashing two-star reviews with callous language, trashing someone's life's work. I have received that feedback many times. Every single one, particularly if it was undeserving, hurts.

While all this is going on, we don't realize that the self within us registers these intentions and actions. When we are unkind to others, we are being unkind to ourselves. The collective negativity of our lifetime influences our present moment's self-worth. The result: I can count on fingers the number of people I have met who have a completely healed relationship with the self.

In my search for worthiness, I realized that I won't find peace in the world unless I am at peace with myself. I'll know how to love the world the day I know how to love myself. Unless I accept my imperfections and recognize them as part of common humanity, I will judge others and remain afraid lest my truth be discovered. I was born to be real, not perfect. To find that peace, self-love, and self-acceptance, I picked my first connection to be with myself.

One of my fellow presenters at the 2024 APA meeting, Professor Julianne Holt-Lunstad, is the lead science editor of the 2023 Surgeon General's Advisory (Our Epidemic of Loneliness and Isolation). She nicely summarized for me how our self-judgments hurt our connections. "When we doubt ourselves, we may engage with others in self-protective ways, closing ourselves off from harm or rejection. In the process, we may be perceived as defensive, closed off, or unfriendly — inadvertently eliciting unfriendly responses in turn. Thus, when we doubt ourselves and worry about rejection, we may be more likely to get rejection, creating a self-fulfilling prophecy that compromises our ability to build strong, meaningful connections."

In the coming sections, I will share a path to shed self-rejection, build self-worth, and nurture self-love. It entails working through guilt, letting go of the myriad self-worth contingencies, and developing a deeper self-compassion, self-acceptance, and self-forgiveness.

Most of all, I'll welcome you to cultivate intentionality — in thoughts, words, and actions. With intentionality, you choose to live by your values. You decide when to change and when to maintain the status quo, because sometimes, choosing not to improve can be a great improvement. In the process, you'll rise in your eyes.

It is essential that you rise in your eyes if you want to rise in the world's eyes. If you don't value yourself, no one else will!

In our time together, I'll also invite you to take better care of your physical body. Likely, you never forget when your child's next meal is due or how long ago your dog had his kibble. Then why would you go over ten hours without eating or drinking anything nourishing? That makes no sense, but many of us do it every day, hurting our being.

Your covenant with yourself includes taking care of the whole of you. Let's do it gently, one step at a time, while not forgetting to keep our compass aligned with our North Star.

6
North Star

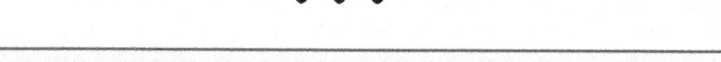

> A hospital janitor saves lives very much like a doctor. Honor the meaning (how one serves the world) not just the means (what one does).

Do you mindfully meet others without judgment, or do you try to figure out their success or influence? At a company retreat, would you give the same attention to the data entry clerk you would provide to the CEO? You know the answers! Paying attention to the resourceful is part of our DNA.

I recently met Stephanie at a conference. A Princeton alum with a brilliant academic record, she is amazingly engaging, humble, and uplifting. Stephanie left a high-paying corporate job to be the best mother for her special needs twins. During the decade she was away, when she introduced herself as a homemaker, at neighborhood gatherings or her husband's work parties, people avoided her like she had the swine flu.

That's just the unfortunate reality. Perceiving time famine and caught in the race to the top, people, particularly the maximizers, invest their moments where they expect the healthiest returns. I say this to state a fact and not present a biased and cynical view of humanity.

As a result, we face a twofold challenge:
1. We get annoyed when people ignore us.
2. When people pay attention to us, we feel that it has nothing to do with us as people; they must need something.

Do you see how that's a no-win situation? To overcome this narrowmindedness, I needed to grow my emotional intelligence and have clarity about my priorities to think bigger than the mundane. Call me a slowpoke, but it took me two decades of research and experience to figure out that searching for and pursuing my purpose could provide me with that growth. This became my second connection.

Purpose: three features

A purpose that can fulfill you and define your life has three core features:

1. It helps others
2. It inspires you
3. It plays out over a long time

A few years ago, I met an investment banker for resilience training. He was struggling to cope with work challenges.

"Tell me more about your job," I asked, not knowing how the investment banking world worked.

"I make money," he said with an expressionless face.

"But you must be doing something, helping someone," I questioned.

"No, I just make money. That's what matters when my team counts the numbers at the end of the quarter," was his flat reply.

Chasing a never-ending goal was accelerating his burnout.

In the past, my instinctive reaction to such a person would have been, *"How selfish."* Slowly, however, my mindset has shifted from considering the person greedy to thinking of him as needy. I feel better equipped to help others with that validating perspective.

Others in the world might have the right to judge him, but in my office, my role is to help while keeping a compassionate heart. The best thing for me to do is to focus on the task assigned to me.

This perspective has brought me peace and improved my healing presence with others. I tried my best to help him see the connection between purpose and his health, happiness, and success, but I was unsure if he was ready to escape the quicksand.

Discover, not invent

Most often, you don't have to invent your purpose; it is waiting to be discovered. Now, it's a different thing if you are a marketing supervisor selling vaping products to teenagers. How likely would your job profile wow members at a high school parent-teacher association meeting?

More than once, I have heard people say that they have an uninspiring job but no way out because they need this job right now to pay the bills and maintain health insurance. In that case, you may have to find your purpose elsewhere, such as engaging in a meaningful altruistic activity during personal time. For most others, consider refocusing what you do with the lens of purpose.

For instance, I could look at my work from two different angles:

1. I am an entrepreneur who builds and sells resilience programs.
2. I work to support the mental health of children and adults globally.

Don't you think the second description will provide me with a healthier sense of self? Once you have that purpose, it'll help to integrate that in your daily life.

A few years ago, while working at the clinic, I had no pep left to see my next patient. I sprinkled water on my face, tried to breathe deep a few times, and gulped a cappuccino — to no avail. When coffee fails to work, you know your fatigue is real.

Then I remembered my purpose, which is to help build a kinder, happier, and more hopeful world for our planet's children. I tried to connect doing my best for this patient with helping children. It so happened that the gentleman was the principal of a high school responsible for over two thousand students. I imagined that if I could help him, I would be helping all those students. That belief was magical. I found the sprint I needed.

Try this for a tedious task. Find a connection between an uninspiring project and your purpose. It will likely become a little less boring.

One of my role models is a hospital janitor who said, "My job saves lives." With that focus, she does her best to clean the hospital rooms so the infection of one patient doesn't go to another. She has found her purpose.

Purpose and loneliness

In 2013, Karen Guggenheim, a communications expert, lost the love of her life, her husband Ricardo, after a brief illness. The loneliness of grief, however, didn't douse Karen's spirit. She transformed it into a passion for bringing happiness to others, founding the World Happiness Summit (WOHASU), which has brought a message of hope and healing to hundreds of thousands of people. In her inimitable eloquence, Karen shared with me how helping humanity helps her own well-being. Karen said: "Helping others has helped me heal and feel less alone. Service is the antidote to my loneliness." People like Karen are the salt of the earth. The research I present below convincingly proves her assertion.

In a thought-provoking study involving 2312 adults, researchers assessed a sense of purpose, loneliness, and other measures. The study showed a positive association between a sense of purpose and social well-being and an inverse association between a sense of purpose and loneliness.[1]

Another study involving 2240 participants showed that the higher individuals attached value and significance to life, the lower their likelihood of loneliness. In fact, scales that measured meaning in life had a more substantial impact on loneliness than social connectedness.[2]

Many people who feel lonely aren't just missing connections with others and themselves. The loneliest among us are also caught in an unlit corner where they can't see the light of purpose.

Purpose vs. process

As you think about the purpose worthy of your lifelong engagement, please parse between purpose and process, for the two are often confused. Purpose is a long-term, personally meaningful goal that helps the world. Process is the steps you take to pursue your purpose. Thus, building resilience programs, writing books, speaking at keynotes, or training trainers is my process, not my purpose.

I know as I advance toward my senior years, I might lose some of my faculties. Yet, I'll only lose the process. No one can take away from me the life-breath of my purpose.

That purpose is your North Star, a trusted constant in your life that will never desert you. Even on days when you can't pursue it with your mind and muscles, you can still track it with your spirit, in prayer. Keeping your purpose in your heart will help you during your most vulnerable moments.

Many of my patients who have well-treated depression or anxiety share that from nowhere, they experience a momentary feeling of emptiness. If not tamed, this feeling becomes stronger, leading to worsening symptoms, including a potential relapse. I have experienced similar symptoms on several occasions. During those moments, one of my go-to practices is to think about my purpose (building a better world for our children) to motivate myself. Alternatively, I pause my day for a few seconds and send good energy to all the children feeling vulnerable today. This simple practice often pulls me out of my languishing moment.

I feel sad thinking about George Eastman, who gifted the world with photography. He was so depressed and in pain during his last moments that he died by suicide. His last words were, "To my friends, my work is done — why wait? GE."[3]

I wish I could talk to him and remind him of the happiness he had brought to people's lives. His purpose, if I am allowed to reimagine with all my respect, was to bring joy to people's lives by helping them capture precious memories. Such a purpose (and not the process) would never be completely accomplished. It will keep you inspired to the very end.

I pray your North Star shines bright on your stellar map.

Looking through the fog for my North Star, I wandered the first two-thirds of my life, touching one meaningless milestone after another. A healthy relationship with the self has awakened me to my purpose — to the enormity of the task at my hand, the importance of emptying the wrong stuff so I have space for the right stuff, and the wisdom of being altruistically selfish. It has helped me embrace uncertainty, embody generosity, and live each day with courage and inspiration so my innately introverted self can find the energy to make meaningful connections with others.

7
Hello Others

> I was much wiser in kindergarten. I knew sharing. I knew how to laugh, hug, love. I did not judge or feel judged. I could forget myself for hours.

"A sixteen-year-old wants to get married to her high school sweetheart. How does that sound?" I asked Kate, an executive who was seeing me for a resilience consult. She was struggling with an unpredictable and somewhat passive-aggressive manager and was considering quitting.

"Not very uplifting," she said. "Unfortunately, so many kids these days are lost. I am worried soon her pregnancy test will turn positive, bringing her education to a halt."

"You are right. But let me tell you the full story. That sixteen-year-old's high school sweetheart has advanced cancer. Doctors have given him three months. She wants him to experience the joy of getting married before he passes away."

After a brief pause, I asked, "What do you think now?"

"That changes everything," Kate said. "I kind of respect her for her fortitude and commitment."

"Do you see how context changes everything? Is it possible your very annoying manager is going through a struggle but can't share it with you?

While that may not be true yet, considering that he has a valid reason might improve your Sunday night's sleep."

"How about I try this with my husband first? But what could be a valid reason for him to leave dirty socks on the floor?!" Kate, a quick thinker, jokingly replied.

"Probably the same reason he forgets his wallet in the refrigerator. He can't get past all the open files in his head!"

Redemptions

I must make some redemptions here. I hope you are not judging me for saying things like, "People, particularly the maximizers, invest their moments where they expect the healthiest returns." I am not being inconsiderate, and certainly do not believe I am sitting on a high pedestal to blurt out these judgments. Judging someone out of context is like reading one page in a novel and calling the story uninteresting.

I unequivocally believe in humanity's goodness. No other species has the depth of compassion or forgiveness that we do. No other species rejoices in helping complete strangers. However, no other species suffers as much emotionally as we do.

I have had the privilege of meeting tens of thousands of people by providing resilience consults and learning the unedited version of their life's stories. Many of these are successful and outwardly happy people with power and glamor. But universally, most of them struggle deep down — with fears, insecurities, absence of love, loss of motivation, and more.

The reason is simple. While we are brilliant at designing skyscrapers and large language models, we are pretty green when it comes to managing our emotions. Our instinctive approach — suppression and distraction — is as effective as running a load of dirty laundry without the detergent. Our minds are also busy with too many open files in our head, decreasing our ability to handle any one issue skillfully.

Chances are you also carry the load of others' high expectations and needs. Expectations raise stress disproportionate to improving performance. Burdened by others' lofty expectations, I often hear people say, "How do I trust people when everyone wants a part of me?" "How do I give what I do not have?"

An executive commented, "I do not get stressed; I give stress." Outwardly aggressive bullies are bullies to themselves. Many, however, aren't aware of how much pain they are causing themselves, having access to a bottle of wine each day to numb their feelings.

Another more self-aware gentleman said, "I'm the only one hurting. Everybody else in the lobby seems okay." After a brief discussion, I asked him, "What if everyone in the lobby feels the same?"

Based on studying well-being, practicing medicine, providing resilience consults, and living life, here is my conclusion: our world is presently overburdened with invisible pain. Many of us yearn to reach a state from which we need no more healing. People are exhausted from being called to act more resilient than they feel. Mental health statistics capture some of it; however, much is silent.

Nevertheless, the world fails to see your pain because, overwhelmed with its own busyness, the world seldom sees you. Unhealed pain slowly erodes your calm and takes away sleep to create a condition that many patients call painsomnia (pain + insomnia). Pain and insomnia feed into each other (pain causes insomnia, and insomnia worsens pain).[1] I have no doubt a considerable proportion of "difficult" people in your life struggle with varying degrees of painsomnia.

Low expectations

Knowing the foregoing (how much people struggle) has helped me lower my expectations of others. I do not expect anyone to give me undivided attention or make efforts to boost my self-worth. If people are annoyed and sensitive, I do not take it personally. If people do not appreciate me, I do not blame them. All of this helps me maintain a healthy relationship with others and is also self-protective, for I am a sensitive soul.

In the past, I got easily hurt. I was the poster child of the "liking gap," which, as the research shows, is people's misperception that others dislike them.[2] For example, after a conversation we might assume that we totally messed up, while they walk away totally impressed. This gap starts very early; even five-year-olds think that their friends don't like them as much as they like their friends.[3]

So, if you promised and didn't call back, I took it personally. If you forgot my birthday, I assumed you no longer cared about me. If you delayed responding to my email or text, I considered myself unimportant. I lacked the courage to be disliked. This sensitivity didn't serve me well while keeping others on eggshells.

The worst part was that what I found annoying about others was precisely what I was doing to them. I procrastinated, forgot people's important events, didn't know how to praise, and didn't acknowledge kind gestures. The list kept getting longer. Then, among many other insights, I stumbled on a useful formula.

A useful formula

Here is the formula:

$H = R - E$ (Happiness = Reality − Expectations).
I edited it to $H = R/E$ (giving even more weightage to expectations).

This is true for my life — the lower my expectations, the higher my happiness. Further, the benefit of working on expectations is even more substantial than changing my reality.

Think about someone who is demanding, noisily complains at the slightest discomfort, doesn't offer any help, and often wakes you up at night. Perhaps they sound a bit annoying. That someone happens to be your three-month-old infant! Do you see how changing expectations can change your perception of the situation?

So, I don't expect a hug right away when it comes to relationships with others. A handshake would do. The story of the handshake is interesting. When warriors clasped each other's hands, they showed that their hands had no weapon, so were not a threat. They called it a handshake because they literally shook each other's hands to ensure no weapons were hiding beneath the sleeves of their arms!

With trust in our society at or near an all-time low, rebuilding trust with the metaphoric handshake might be the first place to start.[4] This applies as much to family as it does to friends, colleagues, clients, and neighbors. Let's rebuild trust to invite love into our space. Love cannot stay in a room where trust has never entered.

But trust is incomplete if it doesn't translate into satisfying one of the most unfulfilled human cravings — the need to feel respected. Respect is the modern language of love. Love and respect share two things in common. One, like love, the best way to earn respect is to give it. Two, respect for the self is essential to getting respect from others. An excellent way to show both respect and love is gratitude. In my view one of the best ways to prepare for a meeting, personal or professional, is to remind yourself why you are grateful to the person you are going to meet. That little reminder can enhance the quality of your every meeting.

Respect and trust, combined with friendliness and kindness, convert professional colleagues into close friends and relatives into close loved ones. In the process, you seed, feed, and weed the garden of your life: seed with the right people, feed with the right values and practices, and weed off experiences that create silos and pull us apart.

You are the gardener who makes the garden happen. Flowers smile and trees fruit when the gardener tends to them well. But who is tending to the gardener? We need fresh thinking to help the gardener through undoing the state of disconnection in our world.

Fresh thinking

Many thinkers on the planet are working diligently to decrease loneliness by bringing us together through changing built spaces, enacting policies and programs that foster connections, empowering healthcare institutions with an understanding of loneliness, and transforming the digital environment to make it more relationship centric.[5] All of these are worthwhile and helpful. But they predominantly address the outer, visible loneliness.

Nevertheless, based on the prevailing theories, over the last two decades, researchers have tested different approaches to stem the loneliness tide: social support, social interaction, mindfulness training, social connection skills, psychological therapies, redesigned physical spaces, technology-based interventions, pharmacologic approaches, and more. The results, as I began sharing in Chapter 1, are mixed overall and mostly only good for the short-term. (Please see Appendix D for more details.)

To be clear, I still believe in the benefit of the above approaches. My primary contention is that their effectiveness critically depends on having a healthy relationship with ourselves. External connections might fail to uplift you when you aren't your best friend. Unless we address our inner loneliness, we won't succeed with trying to come together as a group.

Opposite to that, when you feel worthy through self-love, the world's rebuffs won't matter. Once you realize that, like the moon, you are whole, even though the world can only see a small crescent today, you'll feel complete in yourself, no matter the external rejections. You'll embrace the cyclicity of life, staying humble during the waxing phase and hopeful in the waning phase. That's where I wish you and I walk toward, together.

With the broad framework of three relationships — self, others, and purpose — we will now embark on a three-step journey that will help you shed self-rejection, build self-worth, and nurture self-love through self-respect, self-care, self-compassion, self-acceptance, and self-forgiveness. This journey will entail training your mind through gratitude, compassion, acceptance, forgiveness, patience, courage, purpose, and prayer. Peace, joy, fulfillment, and mental vigor are the natural byproducts of your inner transformation.

Though I don't particularly like the sound of it, let's start with the negative stuff first, specifically self-rejection, which is our first step.

STEP I

SHED SELF-REJECTION

8
Why Self-Rejection?

> Before feeling guilty and rejecting yourself it helps to remember that luck and constraints are not in your control.

Everything was going well for Myrna and Andy, executives at a mid-sized regional bank, until a mid-trimester ultrasound showed that their baby had a hole in her heart. "Most of these holes close as the child gets older," their doctor said then.

Three months into her motherhood, Myrna received an exciting offer to become the manager of a small community bank. It looked like a dream job with a considerable raise. With Andy on board, she took the opportunity and moved her family to a small town. Andy joined a local insurance company until a good banking job came along. It seemed like a perfect peaceful place to raise their daughter Angela but for one challenge — the community had limited medical care, just a tiny clinic with few resources.

Nevertheless, Myrna kept up with Angela's checkups. "Her heart checked out good. No murmurs." Myrna would hear after each visit.

Unfortunately, not all was good. In Angela's condition, a lack of murmurs didn't guarantee a healthy heart. She needed specialized testing, but the closest pediatric cardiologist was two hundred miles away.

By the time Angela turned six, she started missing her growth milestones. She was "congested" all the time. In one of her coughing episodes in sleep, Myrna saw her turning blue. Testing showed she had developed

Eisenmenger's syndrome, a condition where untreated large holes in the heart are no longer curable. "Unless we find a miracle treatment, she will likely make it to her forties," the pediatric cardiologist said.

Myrna was at a loss for how to break the news to Angela. Every time she saw Angela, instead of joy, she was filled with guilt and shame. She started hating her job. But for this opportunity, Angela's condition would have been diagnosed in time, she thought. Countless other what ifs disrupted her efforts at healing.

Not fair

At times in life, despite our best intentions, others get hurt because of our choices. I wouldn't ask Myrna to try and find positive in this situation. She needs validation for her suffering, much before any efforts at education. Validating the pain and providing comfort without forcing meaning starts our healing journey. Asking her not to feel guilty would be unfair and impractical.

But should an eighteen-year-old experience intense self-rejection because two envious bullies posted cruel comments about her looks? Should a middle schooler feel ashamed because someone posted a deepfake embarrassing video of hers?

As you read these lines, tens of thousands of teenagers are experiencing self-rejection for no fault of their own. A constant echo of nasty words from others dominates their self-dialog. Over time those echoes change from second or third person to first person. Then they can't get past this noise for decades.[1] The mean words become their non-erasable life script.

We must find a way to flush these bullies out of our minds because presently, up to eighty percent of women feel that they are not good enough.[2] About the same percentage of professionals believe they do not deserve their success, fearing that someone will soon unravel their incompetence.[3] Eighty percent. That's practically everyone.

This pattern of negativity has many names that describe overlapping constructs — self-criticism, self-disgust, self-hatred, self-loathing, self-condemnation, self-rejection, self-judgment, low self-esteem, low self-worth, imposter syndrome, and more. All of them point to a pervading feeling that I am bad, an underachiever, and thus do not deserve happiness or anything good in life.

Where do these feelings come from, and why are they becoming more prevalent? Why do we speak to ourselves in a language that we would seldom, if ever, use for anyone else? Words like — what a loser, you would never make it, you are an idiot. I can think of seven reasons why.

The seven reasons

Here are the seven reasons that get us stuck in self-rejection, both in its mild and severe forms.

1. Nature's mandate

Some days even the alarm clock's loud blaring fails to wake up your tired brain. One such day, when I got 30 minutes late for an important meeting, I wanted to magically teleport into my office without anyone noticing. The memory of that embarrassment has served me well with my sleep hygiene.

Nature ensures that you remember a negative experience by pouring adrenaline and cortisol into the brain to consolidate those memories. I'm sure you have read how the negativity bias helped our ancestors survive the treacherous ancient world. The consequence of getting caught cheating on your tribe could be a death sentence. That's why nature's default programming makes us feel bad when we hurt someone or even think about acting dishonorably.

But this protective reflex came with a cost. It made us into a paranoid species with a neural system that is deft at catastrophizing.

Inefficient elimination contributes to creating the neural trap. I'm not talking about chronic constipation here, though that can also steal our peace! It's a different constipation — that of thoughts. A rare neurological condition called hyperthymesia can provide a good insight.[4]

Patients with hyperthymesia have the opposite of memory loss — they can't forget anything. I once asked a patient with this condition, "What were you doing on August 28th, 2009?" She paused and shared, "I was in Seattle. My husband and I went to the Space Needle. We ate cheeseburgers for lunch. They ran out of ketchup." She could prove everything with pictures stored in her camera.

While this might sound amazing, people's inability to forget can be challenging. Forgetting frees you from the stuff you forget. Many patients with hyperthymesia experience disabling anxiety because the past negative experiences never fade away. I fear our modern stressors, by repeatedly squirting adrenaline and cortisol in the brain, are creating a biological equivalent of selective hyperthymesia that keeps the negative memories alive.

2. Neural feedback loops

Biological systems depend on automatic feedback loops that can be negative or positive. In a negative feedback loop, the outcome signals the system to stop the process. Thus, eating curbs your hunger, and drinking water quenches your thirst. Negative feedback acts as a governor keeping the system in check. No wonder these loops predominate in most successful systems.

The opposite is the positive feedback loop, where the outcome fuels the very process that caused it. If A increases B and B increases A, then the system can overproduce both for a very long time. A perfectly destructive positive feedback loop is a stampede. The more people run, the greater the panic, which makes more people run. Because of the positive feedback loop, in no time, an orderly congregation can turn deadly.

Only a few positive loops exist in the human body. Lactation is one practical example. Baby's suckling through the release of prolactin releases milk, which prompts more suckling. Another body part where nature has planted a positive feedback loop is in the brain (Figure 4).

Here is how it works. When you think a thought, the brain area hosting that thought gets more blood supply. A greater blood supply brings nutrients that include growth-promoting chemicals (such as the BDNF).[5] The result? Thinking a thought strengthens the brain area hosting that thought. This stronger brain area increases your chances of revisiting that thought and that completes the loop.

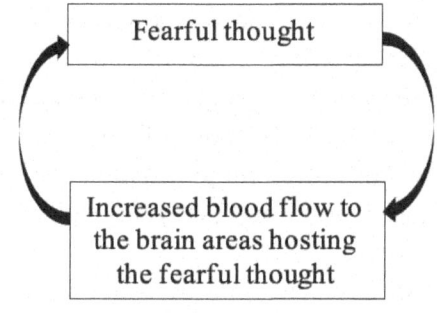

Figure 4. How your brain magnifies fear

Remember the song that got stuck in your head? The more you tried to remove it, the more U-turns it took. Now imagine if, instead of a song, it is a fearful thought. Feeling threatened releases excessive adrenaline. A recurring thought leads to ongoing adrenaline pouring, creating a set-up for a panic attack.

Within limits, the brain's positive feedback loop enables learning (its biological basis is neuroplasticity). Unfortunately, nature hasn't yet figured out how to optimize learning while protecting us from runaway negative emotions.

Those entrapped because of this nature's imperfection are often the ones with the most vulnerable brains — our children.

I feel tremendous sadness when I hear about someone who spent decades of their life experiencing self-rejection because they kept spinning in this loop that started with a childhood emotional trauma.[6] The harder they tried, the more they got stuck, like quicksand.

This process is made worse by the effect of the shadows of our past.

3. The shadows of our past

"It goes way back." Mary, a respected professor told me about her childhood insecurities. "My father lives in my head from when I was a little girl. Every single day, he shouted at me in his drunken stupor — You are a born idiot. You'll amount to nothing. So, I worked hard to prove him wrong. But the more I succeeded, the stronger his voice got."

Mary shared what many of us experience — our repressed past resurfacing, as more of us are now talking to therapists and coaches.

The past can be a shadow, but it shouldn't become our prison. That happens when, starting at a very young age, others start molding you into becoming who you are not. You may have been shamed for disagreeing, not conforming, or crying. Loud laughter was suppressed, and if you didn't obey, you received rejection followed by punishment. Time out in dark places, snatching away your prized toys, canceled playdates, grounding — all of these taught you to repress your authenticity whenever you sensed a power hierarchy.

In this state, your hurts got repressed. Repressed but not healed. That is the part of us we loathe. Once we start loathing our company, we start avoiding ourselves, leading to an inner disconnection. That makes sense because why would you hang out with someone who berates and bullies you all the time?

Further, as we grow up, we discover a competitive world that sends rebuffs. The more we succeed, the greater the rebuffs. Every time you light a lamp, you create a shadow.

Finally, some of us inflict the same rejections on others that we received as a child. It's a no-win situation, predisposing both the perpetrator and the victim to self-rejection.

4. Biases

Let me ask you a silly question. If your hand was to touch a hot pan, what would you do?

1. Withdraw immediately, or
2. Think about the best course of action and then withdraw

Of course, you would withdraw right away. You wouldn't pause to think because thinking is too slow. Thinking also takes effort, particularly when you must think fast. In the words of renowned psychologist Daniel Kahneman, "The most effortful forms of slow thinking are those that require you to think fast."

To overcome the slowness of our thinking, our body compensates with physical reflexes, and the mind with pre-programmed algorithms, also called biases. Biases are unfair preconceived notions for or against something or someone. Biases provide a wormhole from your experience to your conclusion, often making the most negative assumptions (to minimize what experts call the Type II error — the error of missing something concerning if one exists).

Here is how my biases worked while taking a college test:

- I'm sure to get an F on this test (Fortune telling)
- Once I fail this test, I'll be a social outcast (Catastrophizing)
- I seem to be failing all my tests (Overgeneralizing)
- This is all because of my advisor. I should have never taken his suggestion to sign up for this course (Blaming)
- That proctor sure is thinking that I know nothing (Mind reading)

Additionally, I often get stuck with my first judgment (Anchoring) and selectively collect evidence that favors my early beliefs (Confirmation bias). Do you see how our system of biases can suck the positivity out of us?

5. Misclassification

Sometimes we embrace self-rejection in the name of self-awareness. We might feel that focusing on and judging our negatives will help us become more aware, leading to improvement. This is perpetuating a myth and harming ourselves.

A myth is a lie that masquerades as truth. You can't build a life based on myths.

Self-awareness is knowing how well your thoughts, emotions, and behaviors are anchored in your values, and your values in the truth. This knowing is gentle and honest, not harsh and judgmental.

For instance, knowing that I am worse than a crow at singing has served me well in not causing pain to others and embarrassing my family at parties. Perhaps, you know someone who isn't a good singer but doesn't know that! (Psychologists call this the Dunning Kruger effect — an illusion of expertise).

6. The dissatisfied need to belong

One Saturday morning, Sia's new contact lenses were giving her trouble to the point that she had red, irritated eyes. I was concerned about infection. But Sia had just one question — will my eyes clear up by Monday? She didn't want to be the odd one out at school. Blending in was more important to her than the health of her eyes because it was her language of belonging.

You belong when you feel free to be yourself. In belonging, you do not need others' extraordinary kindness. You don't see yourself separate, for you are as much part of the bouquet as any other flower.

Unfortunately, our need to belong isn't presently satisfied for one out of two people amongst us, a number that has been steadily rising over the previous fifty years.[7-8] Even when we are in company, our interactions only infrequently translate to uplifting, nurturing, high-quality connections.[9] For instance, employees consider a whopping 70 percent of meetings a waste of time.[10-11]

When we fail to get respect and love from others, to protect our self-worth, we stop seeking it, perpetuating disconnection. That's how the dissatisfied need to belong leads to low self-worth and loss of self-love.[12]

7. Collective human guilt

We humans are amazing. No other species has evolved to embody Nelson Mandela's forgiveness or Mother Teresa's compassion. We donate almost a trillion dollars to philanthropy every year and hundreds of thousands of our body organs for transplant, many to strangers. Yet, we have skeletons in our closets that some of us worry might fall out if we leave the door open.

We often do not extend our compassion to those in dire need, instead offering support to those who are already strong and can reciprocate. In our need to feed all eight billion of us, we have usurped over forty percent of habitable land, displacing countless species. An estimated ten million animals die from cruelty or abuse every year in the U.S. alone.[13] We are directly responsible for the fastest (sixth) mass extinction event in the planet's history. I would give ourselves a humble but accurate D for how well we have cared for the planet.

Finally, we haven't been kind to our own kind. In the last 2500 years, we have physically and emotionally hurt some of the most well-meaning beings among us. More children and women are enslaved today than at the height of slavery.[14]

What goes around comes around. Our ruthless cannibalizing of resources has hurt our planet and is getting to our physical, emotional, and spiritual well-being. We won't collectively feel worthy until we commit to treating our planet and its inhabitants with greater kindness. We need to expand the Golden Rule.

You didn't choose, did you?

Which of the following did you consciously choose?

1. Your parents or siblings
2. Your race
3. Your country of birth
4. Your genes
5. Your manager's personality
6. Your sexual orientation

None of them.

As we delve into the topic of guilt in the next chapter, I want to remind you that many aspects of your life that influence your mood, well-being, thoughts, and actions are not in your control. Further, you have little to no control over the weather, global economy, government policies, or the minds of the many despots who continue to frequent our planet. So, you won't be wrong to cut yourself some slack.

Only a select few people would strive to decrease your self-rejection or increase your self-worth. Why? Because your low self-worth helps many. With low self-worth, you conform, rarely complain about work conditions or compensation, and have a higher organizational commitment, making employers happy.[15] The submissive you can easily be influenced into fear through exaggerated statistics and lies, making politicians happy. Many people in your social circle and family are glad because you are so "sweet" and adjusting. Marketers are delighted because you buy their products without much questioning when you feel empty.

Thus, almost everyone else but for you is benefited by your self-rejection. I am sure you wouldn't ever volunteer to accept such a deal.

Why not then make a covenant with yourself that starting today, you will replace your inner bully with an inner cheerleader who helps you savor your moments, explores your felt needs, believes in you, and confidently says no when you must? That will help convert inner loneliness into a nurturing inner connection. Bashing yourself won't improve you; it will only give you bruises.

To be realistic, your inner bully won't go away with just a gentle message. You'll have to ride it like a rodeo. Stay in the saddle, play through the dust sparkles, and know that a rip in your jeans is your way to success. With that attitude, you'll ride your way to the bell, beating a feeling that many of us experience starting in our childhood days — guilt.

9
Guilt (and Shame)

> In your darkest moments you may feel like you are a victim. Perhaps you can't stop yourself from going there. But you can choose not to stay there. And that is enough.

I was on an overnight call for my team almost three decades ago during my early medical training. At about 2:30 a.m., I heard a commotion near the central monitoring station. A young patient admitted to the ICU was mistakenly wheeled to my floor and was now in cardiac arrest. I tried to resuscitate him, but it was too late.

Many what-ifs of that night still haunt me. What if I knew he was coming and could be more prepared? What if I was better skilled? What if I had more help? I'll carry the guilt of losing him to the very end.

Through the ensuing years, as my empathy expanded, so did my guilt. I was fortunate to meet many monks, Himalayan sages, philosophers, and scientists. Learning from the masters grew my depth and breadth of empathy, but that was mostly for others. I never considered directing my compassion toward myself. As a result, I became increasingly sensitive without knowing how to reframe my thoughts.

Even minor infractions started bothering me. I showed up more than once at Gauri's school and called her from the class to apologize for being upset at her in the morning. I felt guilty seeing some of my old classmates struggling in life ("Why couldn't I be there for them?"). Even eating my breakfast sandwich was a struggle when my friend's dog looked at me with unblinking eyes, hoping for a few crumbs. Never mind that Mr. Buddy had just gobbled his bacon strips and kibble and was already overweight. I wasn't an uplifting company with so much guilt hanging on my head.

Tabatha

I would have continued like this, moving from one guilt to the next, but for meeting a patient, to whom I am eternally grateful. Tabatha, a forty-two-year-old woman, was in the middle of treatment for stage two breast cancer. Her stressors, however, hardly related to the diagnosis.

She felt guilty about not being able to help her ten-year-old with homework or assist her mom with daily activities. Strangely, her husband convinced her that her cancer was her own doing by living a stressful life and missing her mammograms. So, she even felt guilty about her diagnosis.

A bit angry at her husband, I spent over an hour talking to Tabatha about how her guilts were unhelpful and impeding her healing. "The good people are very good at feeling bad about themselves," I heard myself say to her. "The innocent feels the greatest guilt. Your guilty feelings prove that you are a good person."

"Wait a minute," I thought that evening. "Does this mean that my guilt is telling me that I am a good person?" My best expressions come when my compassion finds its passion. My time with Tabatha was one such moment when I shared an insight with her that I didn't think I knew — at least not until that moment.

I thought deeply about what Tabatha and I discussed, read the relevant research, and then scribbled a few paragraphs. Knowing what I share with you below was tremendously relieving and pivotal in my journey from self-rejection to improving my self-worth. I can't wait to present a summary of that information to you.

Insights on guilt

Guilt, shame, and pride are three self-conscious emotions that originate in our imaginations, describing what we feel others think about us.[1] Here, I'll answer five questions on guilt and shame that helped my understanding and started my journey to overcome self-rejection.

#1. What is guilt?

Guilt is feeling unhappy, sad, or worried from feeling responsible for causing harm. Sometimes, you feel guilty even for an action that may have caused no harm (unearned guilt), such as when you feel like your thinking didn't follow your moral standards. You could also feel guilty from believing you are not doing enough to help.

One example of this is mom guilt. Richa often jokes that "Guilty" is her middle initial. I think it applies to every conscientious parent since a B+ is the best grade I have heard any parent give themselves for their parenting quality.

Here is a comforting thought if your grade is B+ or below. Every parent who worries about being a good parent is already one. This is because the two driving forces for guilt are conscience and empathy. The selfish, greedy, and cruel people seldom feel guilty.

Guilt is ubiquitous; all good people on the planet feel guilty at some point. The key is not to let guilt paralyze you into melancholy. Instead, let your guilt inspire you to become kinder and more purpose driven.

#2. Is guilt the same as shame?

Both guilt and shame might look similar but confusing them is like confusing the plant Boxelder for Poison Ivy because both have compound leaves made of three leaflets. While guilt is a negative evaluation of the behavior, shame is a negative evaluation of the self. Guilt says, "I did bad." Shame says, "I am bad."[2] In shame, you isolate yourself from the rest of the world.

Guilt transiently disconnects you from a part of you; shame rejects the totality of you with no hope of reconciliation. Shame and inner loneliness thus are two peas in a pod.

A research review aptly stated: "Shame drives people to hide or deny their wrongdoings while guilt drives people to amend their mistakes."[3] Below is a table comparing the two (Table 1).[4-6]

Table 1. A comparison of guilt versus shame

Guilt	Shame
Negative evaluation of behavior	Negative evaluation of self
Actionable	Often not actionable
Basis is compassion	Basis is judgment
Externally focused	Internalized
Leads to amending the mistake	Leads to hiding the mistake
Doesn't increase inflammation	Increases inflammation

In shame, your mind becomes fused with the perceived mistake. Like a solar eclipse brings darkness, the negative aspects of your mind eclipse your virtues in shame. You feel this darkness will last forever, not knowing that the darkness isn't real. Instead, light is real. Darkness isn't the absence of light. It is our temporary inability to see the light.

My friend and best-selling author of *The Burnout Fix*, Dr. Jacinta Jiménez, recently shared with me some very wise words on shame. "Shame corrodes the very part of us that believes we are capable of change. It thrives in secrecy and silence, feeding on our fears and insecurities."

When ashamed, self-contempt fills your mind to the brim, it can't take any additional blame. So, you don't accept mistakes even when you are the one who left the banana peel on the floor. Feeling unloved, you try to disengage from the world.

Shame, opposite to guilt, pushes you away from planning and restoring and toward catastrophizing.[7] You feel unworthy and undeserving of love. Thus, shame worsens every single mental health condition,[8] including your risk of self-injury.[9]

Curiously, sometimes shame might outwardly look virtuous. People feeling the shame get overly compliant and hardworking, trying to get over or hide their shame. But this isn't healthy because very likely they simultaneously are accelerating toward burnout and ditching self-care. Consuming excessive calories, loving the couch, waking up tired, and numbing themselves with substances and other forms of addiction are all associated with shame. Sadly, a lot of people experience shame, not because they chose to do something wrong, but because they got trapped in adverse circumstances beyond their control.

#3. What is appropriate guilt? When does feeling guilty make sense?

Guilt is appropriate when your mistake was the direct cause of the hurt, physical or emotional. A complete lack of guilt often accompanies dishonest rationalization or blaming others for personal mistakes. A can-never-be-wrong disposition annoys everyone and perpetuates the wrong action.

Guilt is thus an innocent emotion. It emerges from a desire to be loved. Guilt proportionate to the harm is good for cultivating compassion and future virtuous behavior. Healthy guilt promotes cooperation and selflessness and invokes forgiveness from others, keeping the family or workgroup together. It is a sign of humility.[10]

Appropriate guilt, since it is unpleasant, prevents you from doing wrong. Both empathic concern for others and guilt-proneness decrease the risk of causing harm to others.[11] I don't know how many times I have foregone picking the last cookie, changing the room temperature to my preference, and ignoring a kid selling discounted tickets to a local baseball game because of the anticipatory guilt.

A question that often intrigues me is how much is nature versus nurture. Researchers have been asking the question, is there a guilt gene? We don't have the final answer, but I do believe that our life experiences, particularly our upbringing, interact with our brain's workings (which depend on several thousand genes) to create our "guilt phenotype."[12]

The bottom line is, please do not feel guilty about feeling guilty.

#4. What is toxic guilt?

Guilt is of two types: Benign and Toxic. Benign guilt is proportionate to the situation, leads to a positive action, and fades when the situation resolves. Toxic guilt is a strong feeling of causing harm that isn't proportionate to the problem and is stubborn in its persistence. Toxic guilt doesn't change the past, but it can hurt the future.

Toxic guilt often affects people with guilt-proneness — those who feel guilty for no apparent reason. The guilt-prone people feel guilty all the time for every little thing even when they didn't intend to cause any harm. Often, they carry shadows from their past when the adults around them found it convenient to label them as someone always at fault. They lack a positive nurturing connection with themselves — the very definition of inner loneliness. Feeling guilty becomes the default thought highway in guilt-prone people.

Such guilt leads to low self-worth and self-rejection, impairing relationships, self-care,[13] and performance,[14] and predisposes to post-traumatic stress disorder (PTSD).[15]

You don't need to feel guilty about knocking over a glass of water on the dining table, unless, of course, it wrecked someone's computer in which they had saved the only copy of their family photos. If indeed you carry scars from being in survival mode for a very long time, then you likely need greater self-compassion, self-acceptance, and self-forgiveness. We will come to all of these in the coming sections.

#5. Is shame ever helpful?

This is like asking if smoking a cigarette is ever helpful. The answer might be yes if smoking a few puffs will calm your rage enough to stop you from punching your supervisor.[16] Otherwise, the answer is no.

Similarly, if you have intentionally done something egregious to hurt another person badly, feeling ashamed would be appropriate. But in general, shame seldom helps anyone and doesn't inspire positive change. We hide in shame and feel inflamed inside, hurting ourselves without hope for improvement.

Other symptoms

Other than feeling guilty, what else do we experience because of self-rejection? Here is a partial list of symptoms half of which I have experienced at some point in my past.

Persistent sadness, fatigue, lack of desire to do anything, worrying all the time, social withdrawal, suicidal thoughts, lacking self-confidence, unhealthy relationship with food, inability to advocate for self, avoiding challenges, poor self-care, social sensitivity, hesitating to take compliments, catastrophizing, ruminating on the negative, unable to trust yourself, not enjoying work, and feeling undeserving of anything good in life.[17-24] Many of these feelings worsen your self-rejection, setting up a damaging feedback loop.

Imagine you are meeting four people on Zoom. As you speak, a window appears, and a person talks over you, berating your words and persona. How would you like it? What will that do to your focus?

That person is your inner bully, which feels empowered to raise its voice when you loathe yourself. I'm sure you have seen plenty of combative interruptions on live TV. Never forget you have the off switch if that show runs in your head.

But we feel awkward turning off our inner bully or decreasing its volume. This is because, over time, we start believing the shame voice thinking it means well. We also get comfortable with the negative even though we seek the positive. Let's say you have a choice to seek one of the two feedback options from a colleague.

1. Please share a few good things I am doing at work.
2. Provide feedback on areas where I could improve my performance.

Which feedback would you feel more awkward asking? Most people say it is the positive feedback. We are too afraid to hear how good we are, lest we change our expectations of ourselves and then have to endure the pain of disappointment again.

Further, in our effort to improve, we seldom pause to enjoy how good it already is. I hope you see the vital need for balance.

The above five insights led me to an important next question: how do I tame my guilt and shame? Let's see what you think about my suggestions.

10
Taming Your Guilt (and Shame)

> If today's load feels too heavy, try to pick the load of only the next hour. It might make the load more bearable.

When the human life span was less than fifty years, our immune system's primary task was fighting infections. With increasing longevity, the portfolio expanded. Now, our immune system also detects and neutralizes the occasional cells we all produce that have aberrant DNA. If left alone, these cells can turn against us by becoming cancerous.

Eliminating cancerous cells isn't for the faint of the heart. These cells try every trick to masquerade as normal cells. When the immune system can't tell these destructive cells from the local peace-loving ones, then the bad guys proliferate undeterred, taking down everything with them.

A guilt-laden thought behaves like a destructive cell. It blends in with other elements of your mind until, eventually, guilt becomes a part of your identity. A collection of such thoughts color the lens with which you see the world. Guilt that is not thoughtfully managed becomes a part of your identity. You do not look at the guilt; you start looking at the world through your guilt. In such a state, your efforts at rejecting the guilt risks rejecting yourself, perpetuating the inner loneliness.

Further, previous guilt predisposes you to subsequent guilt, marching you toward toxic guilt and then shame. Shame is thus a consequence of letting your mind simmer in a collection of guilt-laced thoughts.[1]

Two additional processes keep you stuck. One, feeling guilty sometimes feels like being virtuous. So, nurturing guilt might seem like you are doing the "right thing." Two, when guilt dominates your mind, you assume you deserve less, short-changing yourself. Low expectations help dull the stress you might experience with anticipated failures. You thus start seeing guilt as a place of emotional "refuge."

The result, however, is that guilt, particularly toxic guilt, leaves you with low self-worth, hurts your relationships, hampers your performance, lowers your self-care, decreases your courage, and creates apathy. In other words, you aren't thriving; you barely get by. You don't want such a state to become your home. You want to escape this suffocating net to breathe freedom and live with inspiration and courage.

Three lines of thinking can start you on your way to freedom.

1. This isn't guilt worthy
2. I am not the only one
3. I can transform my guilt into something useful

To clarify, we aren't trying to eliminate all guilt. We are striving to tame the unearned and toxic guilt and eliminate the shame masquerading as benign guilt.

Rest assured that just as mud is a temporary state that hides the pure water, you can transcend toxic guilt and shame with effort. Water eventually finds its purity, which is its basic nature. And when you stop pouring impurities, the river cleans itself. That gives me hope.

This isn't guilt worthy

Sometimes the situation might be unpleasant but doesn't warrant guilt. This includes instances where the hurt never happened, the mistake never happened, the mistake didn't cause the hurt, or the mistake caused the hurt but prevented something worse that could have happened.

1. The hurt never happened

You have an office colleague who is unequivocally rude and rigid. You think he doesn't like you and deserves to be badmouthed, an experience you have enjoyed in several of your private dinner conversations with your partner. However, to your surprise, the same colleague gave you the most glowing evaluation on your 360 reviews this week. You now feel guilty about disparaging them. Should you feel guilty?

My answer is no because the hurt never happened. That person never came to know of your thoughts. You also had a legitimate reason for what you said.

Instead of feeling guilty, consider this moment a learning opportunity. Every fantastic person has annoying traits that are part of the "package." Often, people we call bad are good people going through difficult times. Focusing on this learning might help you accept and preserve your authentic compassion for people you find rigid and rude. Trust me, you'll run into plenty of them!

2. The mistake never happened

Let's understand the difference between an error and a mistake. An error is an inaccurate judgment. A mistake is an error that happens when you knew or should have known the right thing to do. For example, if you pull into the wrong driveway because of misdirection by the GPS, that's an error. Similarly, sending an email to an unintended recipient because your autocorrect changed Amit Sood to Admit Soot (my life's story), is an error, not a mistake. But calling me Dammit Slob would be a stretch (a version of my name through a now thankfully extinct autocorrect software). Good people often upgrade their errors into mistakes, while uninformed and not-so-good people maintain a list of people they find easy to blame.

Remember that saying no is not a mistake. You have to say no to others to say yes to yourself. Saying no is often the right and the nice thing to do. Why feel guilty about doing something right and nice?

3. The mistake didn't cause the hurt

A favorite part of my travels is eating new cuisines delivered right to my room through one of the food delivery companies. In one of those gastronomic adventures, I received someone else's order that I had to return. It was late at night, so instead of ordering again, I walked over to the lobby's vending machine. I missed the sign that said, "Caution Wet Floor." I spent the rest of the night nursing my back and a bruised ankle.

Should I blame the food delivery company for my tumble because their mistake started the frustrating chain of events? Probably not. In this case, both a mistake and a hurt happened, but the mistake did not cause the hurt.

It also helps to remember that the mistake might be the final factor, but it often isn't the only factor. It is one amongst countless causes, each of which, if they had acted alone, would not have caused the hurt. This isn't making an excuse. It is stating a fact.

4. The mistake prevented something worse that could have happened

A wrestling match was in progress. It wasn't a fair match because one team had three members on its side, and the other had just one, but a strong one. A nurse, Richa, and I were trying to gently hold down our kindergartener, Sia, for her yearly immunization. Sia hated these shots.

Richa first tried to reason with Sia, who loved her kindergarten teacher. "You need your shots to be in Ms. Cooper's class." Sia paused and stared at Richa. Weighing all her options, Sia said, "No thanks, cancel Ms. Cooper." Stomping her feet, she repeated, "I don't want to go to kindergarten!"

Sensing an impasse, the nurse motioned us for help and before Sia realized, the shots were in. Sia looked at me with the expression, "How could you let that happen to me, Daddy? Not under your watch." I felt guilty the next few days, through her low-grade fever, fatigue, and aches. Gradually, peace was reestablished, and I also got over my guilt by remembering that the shots would prevent her from getting the flu and several other infections.

Sometimes, you have to sacrifice the short term for the long term. The opposite, seeking short-term pleasures that cause long-term harms, is the root of many evils. However, keep in mind that very frequently you won't be a hundred percent sure of what is good in the long term. Impartially evaluate the relevant information and then go with your best judgment, accepting the consequences.

I suggest you pick a personal guilt and take it through these four suggestions. If any of these apply, then it's best to learn from the experience instead of feeling guilty about it.

I am not the only one (common humanity)

Our brain, despite its awesomeness, has some bottlenecks. Two important ones are at the level of attention and working memory.[2-4]

Just as your front door allows only one or two persons to enter at the same time, your attention can entertain a limited amount of input at any moment. That's the reason you can't negotiate with your teenager while reading your company's annual report.

Once the information passes the front door, it enters the working memory of your brain. Working memory is like a foyer, a temporary holding place for information. You call different pieces of information into your foyer to assess a situation. Since the foyer has limited space, you can only consider some aspects of a situation.

Your decision's quality depends on your ability to pull the most critical elements at any time, which as you can imagine, is a judgment call. Remember the last time you said yes to a project that sucked all your energy while offering little gain? When you look back, you can see the reason for failure. But at that time, that reason wasn't accessible, because even if that information was available, you didn't call it into your working memory. History is full of examples of some of the most brilliant people leading their respective Titanic into an iceberg because they were blind to their blind spot.

Further, prolonged or intense stress adversely affects attention and working memory, causing errors in judgment. I once received a surprise excellence award and was asked to give an impromptu five-minute speech. Not only did I forget to thank everyone who deserved a mention, but I also slipped in a few words in a foreign language that only I understood!

Please recognize that these errors aren't unique to you and me. They are a part of our shared human experience. Forgetting important birthdays, completely blanking on your computer's password, or misreading a room isn't a personal failure. It is a limitation of the human brain.

If it comforts you in any way, about seven out of ten people you would consider bright and successful say that they struggle with remembering names, dread when their company upgrades a software, and routinely forget where they parked their car. Working at a prestigious hospital, one of my many fond experiences was having great conversations wandering the parking lot with brilliant physicians while we were both searching for our parked cars.

It's best to learn to laugh at yourself instead of feeling bad, unless, of course, you do not even remember the parking lot where you parked your car. That has happened to me. Good luck with the dinner!

I can transform my guilt into something useful

Discomforting feelings come paired with a change in incentive — to relieve the hurt and prevent future pain. In the words of Dr. Jiménez, "Guilt often signals that we've strayed from our values. If we can learn to use guilt as a guide to realign with what matters most to us, it becomes a constructive force. The key is to acknowledge and learn from your mistakes, make amends if possible, and then release the burden. Remember, growth comes from learning, not from punishment."

While guilt pinpricks may be unavoidable, how you respond to them can change your well-being and life's trajectory over the long term. Pondering over any of the following four questions can help:

1. What did I learn?
2. How do I find more self-compassion?
3. How do I build more compassion for others?
4. How do I make them whole?

1. What did I learn?

The unpleasantness of guilt hides within it a compliment. Listen to its whisper that says, "You are a kind and caring person who wants to feel respected and loved. If you were not, your indifference wouldn't let you feel guilty." Guilt educates you about your sensitivities, pet peeves, and future thoughts and actions to avoid. Walk upstream to discover its origin. You might find things your mind needs to learn to lead a good life in an imperfect world.

An important insight from guilt is that every person you meet, just like you, wants to be respected and loved. People get emotionally injured when this wish remains unfulfilled. Consequently, they start avoiding others to preserve their vulnerable self.

With this awareness, commit to helping others feel worthy. "They like you for who you are. They like you even more when they like themselves in your presence." This simple yet profound realization, when internalized and implemented in daily life, can transform your every relationship.

A useful perspective is to remain a student all your life, so you are open to critique and learning. Here is one simple approach to critique: if not true, ignore it; if true, use it to learn and grow. Keep a thick skin so you do not take critiques personally. If you do, people will stop sharing helpful feedback, which could be a significant loss.

2. How do I find more self-compassion?

Your guilt-proneness and shame both send you a message — your past shadows are showing their ugly head again. You have been repressing them for too long. It is time for healing.

All those messages you heard and internalized — that you are dumb and will amount to nothing — were lies. Someone tried to control your brain by making you feel small. What they said isn't true, it never was.

Look at those memories with self-compassion and self-love. While you can't delete the memories like you can in a computer, you can transform them. See that they are untrue, recognize how they may have affected you, and then focus more on what you see through the windshield instead of the rear-view mirror. We will talk much more about this in the section on self-compassion.

3. How do I build more compassion for others?

Sometimes, we blame and get angry with the very people who deserve our compassion — those who got hurt by us. Our anger helps us feel validated ("It's not my fault, they deserved this"), creating a trap. Staying in your anger's trap could perpetuate unkind actions, seeding future guilt.

Don't let that happen to you. Instead, take charge and ask yourself: How do I transform my guilt into compassion? Perhaps you can focus on others' constraints. People who are busy protecting their vulnerable selves can't bring out their best behavior.

An alternative to compassion is to find more gratitude for the good they bring to your life. One of the best things I have ever said to my daughters is that the energy of their presence has brought good luck to every aspect of my life. Knowing they are a blessing to me without having to do anything helps their self-worth, inspiring them to do even more.

4. How do I make them whole?

A silent, ubiquitous twenty-first-century struggle is feeling unseen. We think nobody cares about our preferences, our pains are normalized and not validated, and our needs are suppressed to quench others' wants. Feeling invisible often equates with drowning in your flood of negative emotions.

Helping others feel seen instead of avoided is an excellent way to overcome your guilt. A few years ago, someone accidentally spilled water on me at a restaurant. They could have apologized and moved on. Instead, after apologizing, unbeknownst to me, they sent a surprise cake to my table. I felt seen by them and now know what to do if I spill water on someone, which I hope never happens!

Shame is flawed

Although science hasn't offered conclusive evidence, I do believe that we all have an innocent, pure, and sacred essence within us. You can choose your preferred name for that essence based on your belief system. So, the classic shame statements "I am all bad" or "I am unlovable" can't be true. If in a bag of oranges, one goes bad, that doesn't mean we need to trash the whole bag.

Similarly, while a part of my mind is a work in progress, it can't be generalized to the whole of me, which is what shame does. Thus, the shame's contention is fundamentally flawed.

That contention for some people is their innate predisposition, which psychologists call "trait shame." People with trait shame feel ashamed, not because they did something wrong, but because some of their neurons misfire to generate shame-related thoughts that the rest of their brain believes. Perception of imperfections, such as their height, accent, sexual orientation, or previous failures might be enough to evoke shame. Often, this process starts early in life, whence the seed of shame is planted in our minds by those we trusted with unconditional love.

Very early in life, when the rushed world around us has little patience and only rudimentary skills to nurture our emotions, we stop stating our preferences. Finding fault in the self becomes our default way of thinking. People who had to pay the price of self-rejection for survival continue rejecting themselves as an adult by developing trait shame.

Notice that like guilt, shame also emerges from a need to feel respected and loved. When the world doesn't meet that need, we hide in our minds to protect ourselves from further injury. The problem is that our mind carries the echo of what it imagined it heard, which is generally negative. We can also be meaner to the self than we can be to anyone else because others give pushback, but no such pushback comes from within us, particularly if we have a shame predisposition.

I wish I could convince a person stuck in this quicksand that their thoughts are nothing but fake self-destructive ogres. Keep in your brain only those people you want to keep in your heart, I want to tell them. However, in those moments, the ogres seem real. Their self-rejection-filled mind doesn't yield easily, leading them to despise every part of their being. Making matters worse, self-rejection becomes a place of comfort. "If I am pre-emptively bullying myself, what worse can happen?"

Expecting people to snap out of their shame, particularly trait shame, is a tall order. A more reasonable expectation is to disentangle the seed of negative thoughts from the rest of the self, which is pure. That's where believing in a core of purity within us comes in handy, a topic I will turn to in Section V.

I have been practicing disentangling for a long time, albeit of a different kind. One of my life's most significant accomplishments is that I'm the go-to person when Sia needs help with her entangled hair ties in her locks. Easing the ties out without pulling hair or causing pain requires skill and patience. So does separating your thoughts of shame that get enmeshed with other thoughts, as if someone bundled them together and sprayed the mass with super glue.

However, once disentangled, at the depth of the froth of shame, you will find a nidus of guilt that is ready to be re-evaluated using the three ideas I shared above: this isn't guilt worthy; I am not the only one; and I can transform my guilt into something useful.

I wish you separate out your feelings of shame from the rest of you, convert the seed guilt you find into compassion and purposeful action, and through this change, feel worthy, develop a deeper self-love, and never experience inner loneliness again.

Self-love and Self-worth

We are slowly moving from the negative pole of our self to the positive. These are not binary feelings. Instead, they are on a continuum. They can also coexist. Despite feeling guilty, you deserve to, and can, keep loving yourself.

A healthy endpoint is where you aren't completely guilt-free but have just about enough guilt to keep thinking and doing the right thing, yet feel good about yourself, and not experience any shame.

As guilt fades into the horizon, you start seeing the glow of two desirable aspects of the self — self-worth and self-love. Although they sound similar, they do have subtle differences.

Self-worth is your belief that you are worthy of belonging, respect, and love, independent of external accomplishments. It is your assessment of yourself.

Self-love is how you translate your assessment into your relationship with yourself. Self-love is thus *respecting, befriending, and nurturing yourself.* Please do not mix it with selfishness, narcissism, or excessively indulging the self. Self-love comes from wisdom, and selfishness from ignorance. We will talk about that much more very soon.

I hope you see the difference. Self-worth is your perception; self-love is your practice. Both self-worth and self-love entail your awareness and connection with your purity. They also involve recognizing and treating your mind's limitations with compassion, acceptance, and forgiveness. Since perception precedes practice, we will start with building self-worth, our second step, and then move to self-love.

STEP II

BUILD SELF-WORTH

11
Knowing Self-Worth

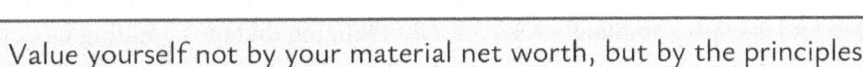

> Value yourself not by your material net worth, but by the principles you embody and the people and purpose you serve.

What would a nine-month-old prefer, a hundred-dollar bill or a squishy toy that squeaks? For them, a dollar bill would be a green paper with squiggly lines that might be fun to chew, but not much more.

When it comes to valuing you, the world is like a nine-month-old. No one else but you recognize that you are worth trillions; you're priceless. Someone else knew that too, perhaps your mother or grandmother. But you didn't believe them then. Now is the time to reclaim your value through building self-worth.

Self-worth, as I mentioned earlier, is your internal belief that you are worthy of belonging, respect, and love, independent of accomplishments. Traditional external metrics such as appearance, achievement, socio-economic status, or popularity do not matter for self-worth.

Interestingly, our self-worth evolves in somewhat predictable patterns over the years. I experienced it firsthand through smiley flowers.

Magic at lunch

One afternoon after I picked up Sia from her daycare, she looked happier than most days. Before I could ask, she excitedly said, "I saw magic at lunch."

"What was it?" I asked.

"The flowers were smiling at me."

I was happy knowing that I was raising a kid with phenomenal self-worth.

When I looked at the literature, it turned out that self-worth peaks in early childhood, and then comes crashing down during the teenage years.[1] Remember how miserable you felt through late middle to high school? That's natural and expected. As we go through college and succeed at careers and relationships, our self-worth improves until it finally plateaus or goes down a bit in our senior years.[2]

The above trajectory is by no means typical. For many, the teenage dip is steep and doesn't completely recover. Not realizing that those pulling us down may be below us in their values, we give them the power they do not deserve. We get entrapped by contingencies.

Contingent vs. intrinsic

Contingent self-worth depends on meeting certain expectations, often demanding we stand out above a certain threshold set by self or others. Researchers often call it self-esteem. Self-esteem is not only unstable; pursuing a high self-esteem is associated with narcissism and bullying.[3]

Intrinsic self-worth, on the other hand, is independent of anything external and is the true self-worth. It inspires humility and kindness, just the opposite of self-esteem.

Unfortunately, the strivings in our society, defined by rivalry, no ceiling, and high expectations, steer us toward contingent self-worth. Out-of-control contingencies can lead to toxic competition eventually leading to failure induced self-loathing. The world that I saw as a child wasn't like this at all.

I grew up in a family of six in a five-hundred-square-foot home on an unnamed street. We had running water for about one hour each day. Some days, we would have no electricity for half the day. We had zero insurance, no social security, and fragmented health care. I wouldn't want to go back to those days, but despite resource constraints, I felt happy and great about myself, partly because I focused on what I had, not what I lacked.

With education, I began climbing the financial ladder. The higher I reached, the poorer I felt because of changing frames of reference. I could now see many more people who were doing much better. When I got a Toyota, I started looking at the Porsche. As technology accelerated, more contingencies crept in through online comparisons — perceived attractiveness, job profile, friend circle, number of social media followers, proportion of five-star reviews.

Then it got sillier. I envied people's mile run time, marathon ranking, frequent flier miles status, and even elite credit card ownership. I would have continued this downward spiral but was thankfully saved by a childhood story that I pondered on as I rewrote it for one of the apps I was developing. It was about a little orphan boy and a fisherman.

The little boy's big true worth

Late on a rainy night, a little orphan boy sat alone on a bridge. He had no friends, no money, and had just lost his pet dog. He felt a pull toward the flooded river beneath him. Just then, an old fisherman passed by. The boy looked the other way. Seeing the boy alone and cold, the fisherman gave him his coat. He also shared his hot chocolate that the boy couldn't resist.

"What's wrong?" the fisherman asked.

"I have no reason to live. I am alone. I just lost my dog. I have no money to buy food."

The fisherman saw an opening.

"What if I told you that you are a millionaire?"

The boy looked at him with disbelief.

The fisherman continued, "I see that you have two arms. How much shall I pay you for your left one? A hundred thousand dollars?"

The boy looked confused.

"How about your heart, your brain, your eyes…The priceless treasure of life within you is worth much more than anything you will find outside."

It took some convincing, but the boy eventually got the message. His priciest possessions were secure within his skin, and they were worth trillions — priceless.

Think about this for a moment. Within you is an essence that is so profoundly amazing that anything material you have or could ever have is trivial. Meditating on this story reminded me of the four-wheel model of my physical-mental-social-spiritual self I had learned at an early age.

The four-wheel model

I can't recall who first taught me this model — my grandmother or my mother — or if I thought about it myself. Simply put, we have four aspects of our being that run our lives: physical, mental, social, and spiritual. You can imagine these as the four wheels of a car.

The physical aspect includes your physical body and all things physical you possess — your home, all your belongings, your vehicle, etc.

The mental aspect includes your cognitive and emotional assets. These are your attention, memory, language, decision-making, feelings, and ability to regulate all these aspects.

The social aspect includes your relationship with yourself, with your loved ones, friends, colleagues, and the rest of the world.

The spiritual aspect is your conscience, your values, and for many, your faith.

In this automobile, the front wheels are the physical and mental, while the rear wheels are the social and spiritual. You can imagine the automobile to be one of three:

1. Front wheel drive
2. Rear wheel drive
3. All wheel drive

None of these is wrong, since no matter the drive, all the wheels are moving. Yet, believing that the physical and the mental aspects predominate risks putting connections and values in the background. I have met many people who have led perfectly comfortable and productive lives with this belief. However, they are less resilient to disruptions, taking a while to recover. Further, almost every person who has done something bad, from simple to horrible, cared little about how their actions affected others or didn't align with humanistic values.

As we mature, we move from front wheel to rear wheel drive. With this change comes the gift of a healthy self-worth. Believing that social and spiritual aspects are the drivers brings out the best in our physical and mental domains.

Eventually, you arrive at an all-wheel-drive model, where you honor every aspect of yourself and others — physical, mental, social, and spiritual — with your values guiding all aspects of your life. You stay busy but do not get overwhelmed. You respect yourself, value yourself fairly, and remember to add appropriate tax on top!

Despite many medical and social odds stacked against me, by the time I became a physician, I started believing that my life's automobile was a rear-wheel drive. This belief helped me treat myself like the prince of my family's five hundred-square-foot estate!

Slowly, after negotiating life's many treacherous terrains, I have come to embrace the all-wheel-drive model. I try my best to treat every part of me and others with respect. I cannot express in words how freeing it is to let go of the need to judge others.

The same applies to not judging the self. Research convincingly shows that the fewer contingencies you place on your self-worth, such as financial,[4] academic,[5] or appearance,[6] the better your mental health and well-being.[7] The reason is simple. Removing contingencies helps you eliminate reasons for self-rejection.

However, it has been all but a smooth ride. Owning an imperfect mind, I have discovered and forgotten my values more times than I care to remember, sometimes for prolonged periods. Why did I forget and continue intermittently forgetting, though less often now? Exploring my failings might help you, just as they helped me.

12
Why Did I Forget?

> Plan for the long term. Live for the short term.

I forgot and continue intermittently forgetting because of two reasons. One, our mind's basic nature is to get distracted and forget. Two, it takes superhuman effort and intentionality to avert the golden cage of our brain's reward network. Here is one example of how it has operated all these years, both for and against me.

At the ripe old age of ten, I had a failed first crush that handed a massive bruise to my appearance-contingent self-worth. I actively avoided girls from there on, which led to my plummeting popularity with the boys, too. With lots of time, I turned to the world's most loyal friend — books.

Bedtime became my book time. After everyone had dozed off at night, I would read with a small penlight beneath the blanket. Becoming book-obsessed rewarded me with academic success, culminating in medical school at seventeen. That's when the magic happened — the neighborhood girls started noticing me.

I reveled in the attention. To clarify, it did not amount to dates and parties. I grew up in a conservative society that frowned upon a boy and girl hugging. All I got was a few extra smiles and more people knowing my name. But that was enough. My brain's reward network had now tasted the apple.

I pushed further into academics, acing every exam and rising to the top of my medical school class and then my entire state. Throughout all this, I met intense competition and won. Each win fueled the flames, which prompted me to compete further.[1] Success was all that mattered.

I got so focused on personal success — my class rank, paper grades, winning debates — that compassion and values went into the background.

I am embarrassed to share an experience I had when I took a test in which I interviewed a patient who was in her fifties and suffered from paralysis of all her four limbs. I focused on getting the most information out of her to top the exam. I had zero compassion for her suffering. I have apologized to her in silence so many times. I so wish I could find her and seek her forgiveness for not "seeing" her at all.

The unbridled pursuit of ego-driven professional success, which further fuels one's ego, can continue for an entire lifetime. In this state, while you are connected to an external goal, you experience inner loneliness for two reasons. One, you aren't comfortable in the silence of your company because every time you seek peace within yourself, you hear the growls of the inner bully that drives you to go out and do more. Two, your connections with others lack authenticity. People are either a means to an end, competitors to be trounced, or a waste of time.

Fortunately, my ego trip was interrupted by a surprise gift — of failure.

The gift of failure

I failed to rank in the top percentile in a crucial national exam, which excluded my entry into an elite program I had coveted throughout my medical school years. What made it worse was that my competitor, my sole source of envy, passed with flying colors. Personal failures are painful; your competitor succeeding while you fail is infinitely more painful!

Failing to secure a college seat in many countries isn't as simple as retaking the SAT. Hundreds of thousands of eager students compete yearly for a few hundred spots. Your chances dwindle with every failed attempt.

That day, I went to the roof of a building to find solitude and sobbed. Getting back onto the highway entailed another year of rigorous work and lots of uncertainty, with my classmates who were now ahead of me enjoying their party banter at my cost. It felt like a tall mountain to climb, thirsty, barefoot, and deconditioned.

As a skilled mountaineer might tell you, climbing a mountain isn't just about physical endurance. It is about your emotional and spiritual strength. It is the mind and the spirit that climb not the muscle.

Constantly competing, comparing myself with others, and worrying about what others might be thinking of me was emotionally and spiritually depleting. I suspect I was clinically depressed at that time, but the concept of seeing a therapist, or a psychiatrist didn't exist in my world. So, I turned to reading philosophy and contemplative texts and attending wisdom discourses that were available to me.

While I didn't have the lucid terminology that I share with you next, it was clear that I had to get past petty comparisons and focus on bigger purpose. I integrate the insights I gained in those years with what I have learned more recently to share a perspective on comparisons as we move from contingent to intrinsic self-worth. I wish I had this insight on the lonely rooftop that day.

13
Our Comparison Instinct

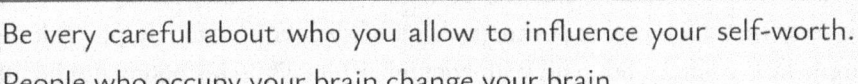

> Be very careful about who you allow to influence your self-worth. People who occupy your brain change your brain.

"The golden rule of medicine is comparison," my medical school instructor often said. "If you want to pick up subtle swelling in the right ankle, compare it with the left." The first step to reading a Chest X-ray is to recognize different normal variations so you can spot the abnormal. Comparison helps us make sense of the world.

But comparison can also create a trap. For instance, envying my colleague who publishes more papers than me or my friend's success with his marketing strategy could put me into a never-ending comparison trap. Much of this process works subconsciously.

A peasant who couldn't afford quality shoes all his youth rose to become a minister. Whenever he would shake hands with dignitaries, he would instinctively look at their feet instead of looking in the eyes. Nice shoes!

Comparison science

Given that comparison sits at the core of our self-worth contingencies, let's explore three key questions:

- Why do we compare?
- What is the nature of our comparisons?

- How can we make helpful and not hurtful comparisons?

Here are my four bottom-line conclusions about the comparison science:
1. Like thirst or hunger, comparison is a core human instinct.[1]
2. We compare ourselves mostly with people who are like us or familiar to us.[2]
3. Comparisons can hurt or help, depending on how we tackle them.
4. Comparisons are of two types: Upward and Downward.

Comparison as a core human instinct

Imagine being a tribal chief fighting another tribe for hunting rights. Misjudging your adversary's strength could be disastrous. Skillful, accurate comparisons were essential for survival, an instinct prevalent in most species.[3]

Like humans, many animals compare not only their strengths but also fairness. In a hilarious experiment, a monkey revolted and stopped doing a simple task when he got paid with cucumber bits while his buddy got healthy-sized grapes for the same task![4]

We compare ourselves with similar others

In a research study, sixth graders based their math abilities on their within-classroom math position and not on whether they were enrolled in a low, medium, or high math achievement class.[5] I'm sure you do not compare your singing finesse with a Grammy winner or creative insights with a Nobel Laureate. Thank goodness, since Gauri once cried when I was singing because I unequivocally annihilated the concept of melody.

Comparisons can both help and harm us

Helpful comparisons get you inspired. Hurtful comparisons predispose you to anger, rivalry, low self-worth, apathy, social awkwardness, malicious envy, eating disorders, and other physical issues. Adolescents are particularly vulnerable to these unhealthy comparisons that are supersized today by social networking sites.[6-8] Unhealthy comparisons frequently lead to self-rejection when you find yourself wanting in a desired attribute.

The two comparison types

Comparisons can be upward or downward. In upward comparison, you measure yourself against someone you think is better than you e.g., comparing your appearance with a famous social media influencer. Downward comparison is the opposite.

Make a guess — which comparison would be more hurtful? I assume you got it right — the upward comparison damages our self-worth the most, creates envy, and prompts us into frivolous activities to boost our self-worth. Social media has hijacked our proclivity for upward comparison, converting it into a driver of worse mental health. Entrepreneurs capitalize on this understanding, integrating this knowledge into their platforms that boost their net worth while simultaneously sending our youth to the ER, having inflicted self-harm.

The preceding tells me that we don't compare because we want to. We compare because we are human. Thus, quashing our comparison instinct isn't feasible or practical. A more helpful approach might be to become more thoughtful about how we compare.

Knowing the basis of hurtful comparisons helped lay the groundwork for me to harness the comparison instinct to our advantage. Let's discuss intensity, intention, and interpretation — three aspects that convert a helpful comparison into hurtful one.

A river's impulse to flow isn't in the river's control. Forces propelling the river originated a long time ago. If you want to work alongside the river, the most straightforward approach is to go with the flow instead of against it.

Thus, instead of letting go of fear, I try to experience healthy fears that will inspire and not deplete me. Similarly, I like pro-social greed, growth promoting envy, and worry that spurs action. I fear I will not use my God-given talents to help others; I am greedy about making a difference, I envy people's creativity in relieving others' pain, and I worry about our present actions that will make the world a less livable place for future generations.

Like the river's flow, our comparison instinct originates in who we are as a species. We can't undo that. Instead, why not embrace helpful comparisons and let go of hurtful ones?

14
Hurtful Comparisons

> Lower your expectations of the people closest to you, so they remain close to you.

Eons before the era of artificial intelligence, someone owned a mirror that could answer every question. That someone was Queen Grimhilde, the beautiful but much-reviled queen of Snow White. Stuck as she was in hurtful comparisons, she asked the mirror only one question: "Mirror mirror on the wall. Who is the fairest one of all?" What a waste of a remarkably useful resource!

Queen Grimhilde made the three classical comparison errors — in intensity, intention, and interpretation. She was consumed by comparing her looks with someone much younger, which resulted in her low self-worth fueled cruelty.

Intensity

Some of us are wired to compare obsessively. Scientists label them as having a high social comparison orientation (SCO).[1] Brains with high SCO have weaker connectivity in their happy areas (the reward network). This might explain their struggle with worthiness and happiness,[2] predisposing them to imposter syndrome.[3]

High-SCO people with luck on their side might taste a lot of success but at the cost of feeling miserable. A very successful colleague of mine got a massive raise, but he was infuriated. When asked he said, "Two people in my group got a bigger raise."

People with a hedonistically driven "I refuse to be satisfied" impulse are tough on themselves and others. When they go inwards, their judgmental self flogs them to do more. Seeking peace and happiness, they go out in the world to pursue pleasure, which often entails splurging. Their splurging comes at the cost of depleting rainforests, heating oceans, and accelerating the ongoing sixth mass extinction, estimated to be a thousand to ten thousand times higher than previous natural extinctions.

The moment they close in on an egocentric goal, they kick the goal post farther. They don't do well with failures, a skill that's essential for youth today. In my work with people from different professions, I uniformly find that a small-town electrician has better self-worth than a successful startup's CEO.

Intention

Social media researchers talk about opinion-focused versus competition-focused comparisons. Comparing to learn others' opinions can be helpful. For instance, staying a lifelong student in relationship intelligence, cooking skills, and lowering your carbon footprint helps you keep growing while helping the world stay livable.[4] But the moment competition creeps in, anxiety and depressive symptoms follow,[5-6] trailed by other scourges like low self-esteem and poor lifestyle choices.[7]

Most of these harms happen with the upward comparison, which gets our impressionable minds inundated with stories of perfection and success that don't match our reality.[8] Unfortunately, the most affected are often children and adults who lacked loving caregivers as a child. A not uncommon consequence is self-numbing to addicting agents or experiences, which pushes them into a downward spiral.[9]

Smriti Joshi, Chief Psychologist for an international mental health platform, knows fully well how upward, competition-focused comparisons shackle us to seek constant validation from others and ourselves. She shared with me the following words that encapsulate her learnings from thousands of her clients: "Our sense of self-worth is often clouded by the harsh inner voice we've internalized from the critical voices around us. Over time, these voices blend into our own, convincing us that our worth is conditional, dependent on perfection, or tied to external validation." Joshi reminds us that self-worth contingencies are present across the world in widely different cultures.

Interpretation

Does your comparison interpretation lead to admiring others or thinking small of yourself? A uniquely harmful comparison is one focused on appearance. We compare our ordinary present with someone's carefully curated best self. Our appearance-focused comparisons, when excessive, become verdicts of personal unattractiveness, hurting body image and mental health.[10-13] Admiring beauty doesn't mean you belittle yourself (or seek to forcefully acquire what you admire), but that's where our instincts take us.

Admire beauty like you admire the full moon — with no envious thoughts and no impulse to own. I wonder how many immoral, cruel, and criminal acts we might be able to avoid on our planet if we transform our selfishness and immaturity into innocence and respect. Having said that, there is no need to be embarrassed if occasional immoral imaginations intrude your thought stream. Every person's brain produces them. Just don't act on them.

Here is what keeps me up at night. Our youths' overly excitable reward network makes them extremely sensitive to personalized social feedback, both positive and negative. Social media designers are capitalizing on young people's sensitivity to social feedback and rejection (such as the number of likes and follower counts). They are working to hijack our children's brains by latching onto their comparison instinct, feeding them content that preys on their vulnerable brains. The resulting hurtful feelings range from malicious envy, low self-worth, and depressive symptoms to thoughts and actions that could lead to self-harm or harming others.

It doesn't have to be this way. We can harness the comparison instinct to help us grow our self-worth while becoming more effective at building a better world. Let's explore the art of helpful comparisons in our desire to make that wise choice.

15
Helpful Comparisons

> Sometimes it helps to notice the yards with more weeds to enjoy yours with fewer.

A perpetually open window on my phone is the photograph of the pale blue dot — Earth's February 14th, 1990, selfie taken from 3.7 billion miles away by NASA's Voyager 1. In the vastness of space, our planet is a barely visible tiny dot, less than a pixel in size buried in bands of sunlight.

This picture helps me zoom out, bringing me to a place of equanimity. It puts all my strengths, weaknesses, achievements, and failures in perspective. I transcend my comparison instinct. Everything that seemed big to my little mind starts looking appropriately small. I find peace again, remembering the message I have on my refrigerator door: *I am enough. I have enough.*

I wish I had seen that picture before sending Gauri from a small-town public school to a world-renowned college. I had many sleepless nights wondering how Gauri would cope with the pace and the inevitable imposter syndrome.

About six months into her experience, I asked her how she was doing. Attuned to my worries, she was very forthright. "Great! I see so many super-accomplished people, but I realized there's no point comparing myself with anyone, Dad," she said. "Everyone has their path. I'm just happy and proud of their success." Seems like she had read this chapter even before I wrote it!

Helpful comparisons have three characteristics: they are fewer and less intense, they tend to be more opinion versus competition-focused, and they help you feel better about yourself and others.

Fewer and less intense

I have an invitation for you. This week, let go of all upward competition-focused comparisons. Celebrate others' success instead of thinking their achievements are undeserved, considering why it isn't you, or feeling envious. Psychologists call celebrating others' success, capitalizing.[1-2]

In a cleverly titled study, "Will you be there for me when things go right?" researchers found that celebrating people's good moments had a more significant positive effect on relationships than being there for them during moments of struggle.[3] A person with whom you can share your happiness without a fear of envy is your true friend.

Here is an example. If someone got their dream job, here are three possible responses, among others:

1. "I'm so happy for you. You completely deserve what you got and some more. When is the party?"
2. "I, too, got that job a few years ago but didn't take it."
3. "They work you so hard and only pay pennies. I would never work in such a toxic culture."

The first response is the obvious best choice. Ideally, you want to authentically bring this response without the need to force yourself. Authenticity is powered by an abundance mindset instead of a scarcity mindset. The world has enough and more for all of us. If someone else has an excellent opportunity, that doesn't mean they have usurped something from me. An abundance mindset is the nature of a simple, innocent mind, which is the happiest.

Dialing down comparisons doesn't mean bypassing the pursuit of excellence or saying no to opportunities. It is the opposite. With a more accessible mind, you can more easily focus on your abilities, strengths, and gifts. Instead of getting better than someone, focus on becoming the best version of yourself. You'll find more courage to take the right risks. You'll learn to savor your success. While continuously improving, you'll keep recharging by enjoying how good it already is.

Frequent recharges are essential to prepare you for a marathon, which is life. Life is a long journey, not just the next quarter or capital raise. Talking to young entrepreneurs at the Forbes Under 30 forum, one of my key suggestions was to stop running a marathon like a hundred-meter sprint. Many do so because they see supremely confident fellow runners finding short-term success with the sprints.

What they don't see is the rapid buildup of exhaustion. Often, we only see the sprint, not the exhaustion, because sprints are loud and visible, while exhaustion is silent and veiled.

Opinion-focused

Thoughtful comparisons inspire you to work toward honing your skills instead of wasting time feeling dispirited.[1-2] For instance, research shows that comparing to learn from others can help you:

- better manage fears[3]
- improve your parenting skills[4]
- stick with an exercise routine and positive health behaviors[5-6]
- manage regrets better

Such helpful comparisons are more accessible for adults with a secure self-worth. But I worry a bit about our children.

One of my worries is the kind of role models our children meet through media. Children understandably get confused when ostensibly mature people behave worse than unruly apes. Children get even more baffled when millions applaud crude behaviors like backbiting, lying, insulting, hating, and name-calling. Worse, when children see their high school valedictorian pitch drunk making a fool of herself with no adverse consequences, they get conflicted. What's right and what's not? Why shouldn't I break the rules and have the time of my life? Why should I be nice?

I also had similar conflicts growing up. Fortunately, I learned a lesson I recently shared with Sia when she asked me about a rude classmate. My response was, "Every person can teach you something. Some teach you what to do; others teach you what <u>not</u> to do." It is essential to see rowdy behaviors as a model of what not to do since our children are bound to see stuff we don't want them to see. We can't raise them in a sanitized world.

My favorite is the previous example — noticing others' destructive behaviors to learn and grow. I have used downward comparison many times to recover from my goof-ups. Whether forgetting a doctor's appointment or spilling milk on the dining table, recognizing that you share these glories with many other co-travelers on this planet can be healing. The day you manage to char your pizza you don't want to be inspired by your neighbor's cooking finesse. You want to hear how they created Fourth of July-style fireworks in the oven.

What are you hungry for?

"My twenty years of work is melting away in front of my very eyes and I can't do anything about it." Maurice sat in my office; his ears turned crimson red. He had built his software company, person by person, and now in the throes of competition, he was fearful they wouldn't survive another quarter. Paralyzed by fear, Maurice couldn't go to his office for a week.

"I want to liquidate my company while there is still some value," he said.

I leaned forward, touched his forearm, looked into his eyes, and said, "Maurice, I think you are running away from fear, not chasing meaning." He thought for a while and then agreed, "You are exactly right. But I was never like that."

What followed was a wonderful discussion about how fear and meaning play different parts in our decision-making and how he can build the right mindset before taking important actions.

Maurice ended up selling his company, but not right away. He revamped his product offerings to maximize value, looked at the next opportunity that could use his expertise and that of his employees, and then took the call.

During our meeting, Maurice wasn't hungry for validation. He needed insight and inspiration. Knowing what others or I are hungry for is extremely helpful in making the proper comparisons in a situation.

For example, when Richa struggled with a difficult friend, she didn't need any insight. What helped her was hearing that the person had annoyed a lot of other people as well (validation). Similarly, validation alone wasn't enough when one of my students failed an exam. He needed to improve his studying style, so comparing his style with others who were successful helped.

On a lighter note, I haven't ever made more successful attempts to inspire anyone with upward comparison than with Simba. Every morning, when he takes his time, I inspire him with how good all the neighborhood dogs are.

"See, Moni gets the job done in 30 seconds. Did you hear how Buddy obliges right when he arrives in the yard?" Inspiration works like a charm with him. No species is exempt, and no age is too soon!

No age is too soon

At what age can we start teaching our children the art of healthy comparisons? The earlier the better. Sia saw flowers smiling at her in her preschool years. Now, in seventh grade, she already finds gratitude cringeworthy!

Research supports Sia's evolution. As I shared before, we feel the worthiest in early childhood. By early double digits, our blues start getting bluer. Adulthood gets a little better, but past middle age, we again struggle.[8-14]

Just as a higher peak bone mass at a young age protects you from older age osteoporosis, similarly, children with higher intrinsic self-worth at a young age have better mental health when they get older. Keep in mind that a review of 192 studies involving over 700,000 people showed that nearly 50 percent of mental health disorders start by age 18 and 62.5 percent by age 25.[15] No wonder, in my resilience consults, the single most common concern individuals raise is about the next generation.

In the last five years, I can count on my fingers the number of people who said their kids are optimally happy and nicely connected with family and others. That's why, whether it is a keynote for an audience of 500 or an individual resilience appointment, I share the importance of helping our children develop intrinsic self-worth every single time.

Many of the ideas I share in the coming chapters apply to you and the youth in your life. Most of these converge to progressing onto the next stage of your commitment to self — moving from healthy self-worth to deepening self-love.

Don't take the bait

"Don't take the bait. Don't take the bait. Don't take the bait." I heard the voice ringing in my head. In front of me was a medical student who I thought was rude and self-serving. She was upset about why she wasn't the first author on a paper in which she had barely contributed. We had several senior professors on the team whose contributions were much more substantial. No way could I supersede them.

"I think you are biased against me," she growled. "You should have told me before I started that I won't be the first author." Ten years ago, I would have easily lost my cool. *"You have no idea what you are talking about. Go read the authorship guidelines. You might not even qualify to be an author. So, just be grateful for what you are getting. And this is no way to talk to your professor."*

But now I have better self-awareness and self-worth, which helps me not lose my cool in front of a misinformed person. When you see an angry person as someone struggling with misplaced expectations, instead of reacting to their words, you naturally lean toward compassionate validation and education.

"I hear you," I said. "Would it be OK to read our institutional authorship guidelines together?" She agreed. We read the guidelines, which, after a bit of back and forth, were followed by her apologies.

Some nurturing words were now in order since she was visibly embarrassed, and I also wanted to convey that we still had a good rapport. I have three personal relationship rules:

- Have a high threshold to give up on people
- Always keep communication channels open
- Never create enemies

"Thank you for trusting me with your emotions," I said. "Your passion and energy will be invaluable as you get busy protecting your patients' interests." I pray I left her with a positive and nurturing connection with herself.

A healthy self-worth that translates into self-love can protect all of us.

STEP III

NURTURE SELF-LOVE

16
Understanding Self-Love

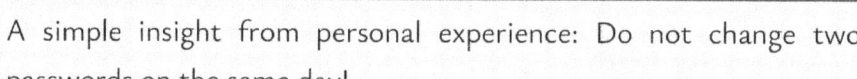

> A simple insight from personal experience: Do not change two passwords on the same day!

I love paneer tikka masala. I also love sleeping in, freshly brewed coffee, a good parking spot, authentic praise, warm hugs, and that relaxed feeling after a good sneeze. These experiences provide me with pleasure, validation, and sustenance, so I *desire* them.

The second shade of my love is *caring*. I have a special place in my heart for my wife, children, parents, siblings, friends, neighbors, patients, and students. I love them all even though at times they may be annoying. Who said caring is always fun?!

In my caring journey, a few years ago, I discovered a previously unvisited corner in my heart — for myself. I never thought I needed that space, until a kind, beloved, and charming student in my community chose to go back to the angels to seek the love they felt the world would never give them. Confused and sad, I looked around to make sense of their pain. That's when my eyes opened to a pervasive lack of self-love. Many intelligent, wonderful people I asked felt self-love would be indulging. People confuse self-love with selfishness, narcissism, or fueling one's ego.

Self-love, however, isn't doting, pampering, or spoiling yourself, even though I find nothing wrong with doing that occasionally. Self-love is waking up to the idea that you are a diamond that may be mistaking itself for an ordinary piece of carbon. No amount of love from others will reach you if you do not love yourself.

Here is how I define self-love: *respecting, befriending, and nurturing yourself.* Let's look at each element one by one.

Respecting

Respecting yourself is valuing your feelings, preferences, and rights. Your self-respect is unconditional, beyond skills or accomplishments. In the words of Dr. Seuss, "A person is a person no matter how small."

Unconditional respect means you feel equal to all. Neither superior nor inferior, just equal. Equality is freeing. When you feel superior to someone, you are bound to feel inferior to another, and vice versa. Thus, feeling better or worse than others isn't a stable, peaceful state. The best mindset is egalitarian. I love pondering the Italian proverb, "At the End of the Game, the King and the Pawn Go Back in the Same Box."

Feeling equal, however, isn't easy, given our instinct to compare attributes we find meaningful. That's where thinking about your essence, the best version of you untouched by the world's blemishes, one that is "beyond comparison," can help. Assuming the presence of absolute purity within everyone makes us all equal and profoundly related to each other.

Your purity never falls from grace, you aren't vulnerable to temptations, you feel confident in setting boundaries, and you aren't a people pleaser. Your essence doesn't suppress desires or creates turbulence if minor preferences are unattended.

While you can't see your purity with your bare eyes, you can feel it when you get past your mundane identities. One such moment for me was at a grocery checkout line. Ahead of me was a very social baby mischievously smiling at me. I smiled back; she beamed even harder. Our silent communication continued for the next several minutes. All my identities ceased. My job profile, unpaid mortgage, country of origin, medical diagnoses, or unanswered emails didn't matter. The baby helped me experience my essence.

I pray we all feel our purity daily through experiences that help us transcend our worldly identities. We will never fall from grace once we connect with ourselves beyond our mundane descriptors. Our friendships will be authentic, deep, and enduring, with others and ourselves.

Befriending

The word friend originates from *frēond* which according to the American Heritage Dictionary means "to love, like, honor, set free". You seldom feel lonely in the company of a good friend. Finding a trusted friend within the self is not only wise but essential in today's world, where no matter who you are, someone in the world rejoices in shooting sharp arrows at you. Befriending the self helps you wear a Teflon vest that repels these arrows. It also enables you to find good friends in the world.

Good friends embrace your innocence and vulnerability. They help you be compassionate, accepting, and forgiving of yourself. Lucky for me, I found a role model of friendship where I was least expecting it — on a street in Chicago.

A few years ago, while walking in Chicago downtown, I saw Bob, a homeless man, playing with Goldie, his golden retriever. Goldie didn't care that Bob was missing half his teeth, coughed every time he laughed, and fed him leftovers retrieved from garbage cans. If I read Goldie's mind correctly, these are precisely the things he loved the most about Bob. Goldie would rather play with Bob by a dumpster than be in a mansion with someone who labeled playtime as "unproductive."

I want to be my Goldie. I want to feel good without needing to feel successful. I want to hold myself today as I was once held by someone who loved me unconditionally. I want to feel the compassion behind my sadness. I want to be happy in my presence doing nothing. In failure, I want to tell myself what I will say to my best friend — I believe in you; you've got this. I know if I treat myself like this today, I will nurture the world with the same energy tomorrow.

Nurturing

Almost a decade ago, Richa and I planted two holy basil plants in a small pot in our home. After growing to six inches tall with about twenty leaves, the plants stalled. Dissatisfied with the progress, we got two big planters (80% off!) to give our basils more space. We also moved them closer to the window for more sun. Ten years out, the plants stand three feet tall and have about two hundred leaves each. Nurturing works.

Presently, we humans aren't nurturing our bodies and minds for optimal well-being. The results speak for themselves — we spend the last ten years of our lives with a significant chronic illness.[1] Many scientists, some of whom are my close collaborators at the Atria Academy of Science and Medicine, are now moving past prolonging our lifespan, focusing more on our health span — the number of years we stay healthy.[2] An essential part of self-love is nurturing your physical self through a healthy diet and physical activity so you stay well and full of vigor until the end.

Fortunately, we know precisely what to do. Eat a predominantly plant-based diet emphasizing variety and high-fiber whole foods. Prefer water over juices and avoid processed foods and refined sugars. Limit red meat intake and make sure you are well-hydrated and micronutrient replete.

Yet, while we might fill the premium gas in an expensive car, we let junk, microplastic-rich food get into our priceless physical bodies. Consider making one change from a few below this month and stick with it for the rest of the year.

1. Increase plant-based food by 10 percent.
2. Have at least one high-fiber food in each meal.
3. Stay well-hydrated (an excellent way to measure this is by having light-colored urine).
4. Decrease processed foods by 10 percent.
5. Increase micronutrient (vitamin and mineral) rich food.

The fifth one is my favorite — increase micronutrient rich food. Before eating something, consider whether your food has adequate vitamins and minerals. Of course, sodium chloride (common salt) doesn't count as a mineral!

Nurturing the self also includes keeping yourself agile, giving your brain and body adequate rest (through sleep, meditation, and other mind-body practices), and having the right personal formula for productivity. Regarding sleep, I can never forget what I read in a research study a few years ago: the lab model of an older brain is a young brain that hasn't slept well. If I do not want my brain to be biologically twenty years older than my chronological age, then I must give it the rest it needs and deserves.

What is productivity?

I often joke that the more I prioritize my well-being, the more hours I work. It has reached a point where I now work twenty-two hours a day. How could that be, since I am not a dolphin who can remain awake all 24 hours, having mastered the art of letting only half of her brain sleep at one time?

The answer is in rearranging the math. I have changed my productivity equation. The old equation was the standard definition, which looked at tasks accomplished for the time invested. Evaluate my new equation and see if you agree with it.

Old Equation

$$\text{Productivity} = \frac{\text{Tasks}}{\text{Time}}$$

New Equation

$$\text{Productivity} = \frac{\text{Tasks} + \text{Recreation} + \text{Workout} + \text{Connections} + \text{Rest}}{\text{Time}}$$

Productivity isn't just doing the urgent; it is accomplishing the important. While the world may have its preferences, I like the new equation better because it includes much more of what I consider important. Thus, I count sleep, time spent socializing, workout, and recreation, as productive time.

One of my silent teachers is the cornfields of Minnesota, many of which are five minutes' drive from my home. The corn fields rest in the winter to sprout in the spring. They have taught me the value of rest as an active part of my life. So, I am not lying when I say I work twenty-two-hour days!

What doesn't count is my worrying time, time spent thinking junk thoughts, and frivolous web surfing (with one exception — online shopping). I love buying practical, cute, and yet inexpensive gifts for others. Giving a good gift is great, not only for your relationships but also for your heart and digestion. That's because of the strong connection between your three brains.

Your three brains

Yes, you do not have one or two, but three brains. The first one of course is the big brain in your cranium. It is a network of about eighty-six billion neurons. The second smaller brain is in the GI system from the beginning to the end, made of about one hundred million neurons. The third, littlest brain is in the heart, with about forty thousand neurons.

These three "brains" have their independent lives and responsibilities, yet are closely interconnected, influencing each other's performance. That's why, when you feel stressed, you often have symptoms involving the brain (memory loss, distraction), the heart (palpitations, dizziness), and the GI system (heart burn, indigestion).

Your gut might not philosophize, but it feels, sometimes even faster and smarter than your brain. I trust and respect my gut's honest and intuitive gurgles, occasionally more than my brain's biased and intrusive pontifications.

Your gut, heart, and brain, all get healthier when you love yourself, have a positive self-worth, and feel connected to others. In the process, you also activate your anti-inflammatory genes. All of this prepares your body for longevity, not just the lifespan, but also the health span.

Tone matters

Food, praise, and play — these are three good reasons why Simba gets out of his crate every morning. Sometimes, to entertain friends and family, I take advantage of his inability to fully understand the nuances of human language. In the most loving way, stroking his belly, I would say, "Simba, you won't get any treat today." "Simba, you are a bad dog." "Simba, today no one will play with you." He would still be there wagging his tail, tongue lolling out, happy that good things are coming his way.

On the other hand, if I say in an admonishing tone, "Simba, you are the best dog ever," he would cower down, scared.

What you say is important, but how you say it is even more important. Tone matters, sometimes even more than the words. When you speak harshly to yourself, you stimulate the same brain areas that activate when the brain experiences bullying.

A simple practice to become kinder in self-talk is to smile with your eyes during the empty moments of the day, also called a Duchenne smile. Eyes don't lie. While you can smile with your lips and still be upset, you'll find it very difficult to be a self-bully while smiling with your eyes.[3] An added advantage is that people like you more when you sport a Duchenne smile![4]

Self-love, as we just saw, includes taking care of both your body and your mind/brain. In the words of Arianna Huffington, founder and CEO of Thrive Global and an admired colleague and friend, "Life is challenging enough without adding our own self-criticism into the mix. It's that voice I call the obnoxious roommate living in our head, the voice that feeds on putting us down and strengthening our insecurities and doubts. We all live with this voice, but the times it comes out the most is when we're tired, stressed and run down. That's when we're most likely to doubt ourselves, most likely to react emotionally and when our perceptions — of everything, including ourselves — are at their shakiest. One of the ways to silence that voice is to take care of ourselves by taking time to recharge. This creates a more robust inner immune system that prevents that voice from breaking through and wreaking havoc. So, prioritizing our well-being makes us more resilient not just physically but mentally as well."

Heeding to Arianna's nudge, lest we forget to pay attention to our body, I wish to dedicate part of the next chapter to reminding ourselves of the importance of nurturing your most precious and sacred temple — your physical being — to enhance your shelf life (I mean longevity)!

17

Say No to Life Limiters

> Here is the essence of thousands of well-being and longevity studies: Adding life to your years adds years to your life.

U.S. healthcare expenditures are nearing $5 trillion, inching closer to twenty percent of the GDP. Yet, most health outcomes have little to do with healthcare.[1-2] North of eighty percent of people's well-being depends on their behaviors, socioeconomic factors, and physical environment. Researchers call these social determinants of health. A few specific aspects include housing stability, food security, physical safety, financial health, community support, employment, education, substance use, and access to the outdoor environment.

Some of these are actionable at the individual level. While you may not be part of your city's highway redesign committee, you are a master of your own being. So, while talking about self-love, I would be remiss in my duty if I do not share with you a few modifiable factors that creep into our lives from unguarded corners and increase our risk of early exit from this planet. A positive nurturing connection with oneself includes treating our body as a sacred gift and taking good care of it. Please pick at least one of these and try to make some improvements.

Five life limiters

1. Prolonged sitting

A recent study of over 450,000 people showed that those who mostly sit at work have a 16 percent higher mortality risk.[3]

Called the "sitting disease," prolonged sitting literally starts melting your body. Your muscle mass decreases, your bones begin leaching calcium, and your blood sugar and triglycerides go up, all increasing the risk of diabetes, cardiovascular disease, and cancer.[4-6]

After an hour of sitting, get up from your chair and take a brief stroll, or if you can, do a few squats, pushups, or jumping jacks. Combine physical activity with engaging your senses, such as listening to music, appreciating art, or noticing colors in the outside world. Exceptions might be while watching an opera performance or during prolonged dental cleaning!

2. Excessive fatigue

A study of over 18,000 participants over 16 years showed that a high level of fatigue was associated with a 40 percent increase in mortality.[7]

Please allow me to wear my internal medicine physician hat to lecture you for this paragraph. Fatigue has three leading groups of causes: medical, muscle, and mental. Muscle and mental fatigue are often from overexertion and generally get better with rest. My focus here is medical fatigue, which could mean many different things, particularly if you don't feel refreshed after a good night's sleep. Is your thyroid ok? Are you anemic? Are you low on iron? Are you vitamin D replete? Do you snore and could have sleep apnea? You also want to ensure your electrolytes, kidney functions, liver, heart and lung functions, and adrenal glands are good. See a good doctor to get help for persistent fatigue.

Fatigue isn't nature's imperfection. Fatigue helps you disengage before injury. By causing fatigue, nature signals you to take better care of yourself and look out for trouble in its early, curable stage, much like the lights on your dashboard that alert you to your car needing repair.

3. Emotional suppression

In a study involving over 700 people, those who regularly suppressed their emotions had a 35 percent higher mortality risk.[8]

Suppressed emotions fester like a deeply seated wound covered by a band-aid. When you are on stage performing in front of an audience of 400, suppressing fear might be appropriate. But for the long-term, go upstream on your emotions to find and heal the original hurt.

One of the ways suppression multiplies your hurts is by seeding ruminations that create an ongoing echo in your brain. Opposite to that, sharing with someone well-meaning fades the echo and divides the pain. Thus, a powerful way to minimize emotional suppression is to connect with someone kind who won't judge you as they listen to your struggles. That person could be a friend, a loved one, a professional, or even your diary.

Not suppressing emotions doesn't mean unleashing explosive anger. After a nasty rage episode, your risk of heart attack goes up several fold for a few hours.[9] So, emotional suppression and explosive anger are both hurtful.

Understanding mental health has helped me better regulate my emotions. Mental health is a combination of *authentic positivity and contained negativity*. A healthy mind doesn't delude itself into unbridled positivity. It relies on truth. It knows that even after the thorn is removed the finger will keep hurting for a while. A healthy mind also has a generous space for negativity. Situation congruent negative emotions that do not lead to runaway anxiety, sadness, or rage are healthier than suppressing those feelings. In other words, our mind is in greatest harmony when it can access and accept the *truth*.

4. Hopelessness

A study of over 70,000 participants showed that optimism was associated with 29 percent lower mortality.[10]

Think of the moment you were born. You had zero control. Yet, your presence today is proof that it all worked out. You have much more control today compared to the day of your birth. So, why won't it work out now? Roll the dice in your favor by staying hopeful.

Hope is the expectation of a better tomorrow. Hope knows the sun will eventually rise even though the horizon might be completely dark right now. It always has and always will. Hope remembers that all traffic jams ultimately clear, the boring meetings end, and babies grow out of diapers. Hope doesn't get bored watching the slow-moving tragedy you can't escape because of social pressure. Instead, hope zooms out into a fantastic future or a beautiful past.

During despondent moments, please remember that most of your fears have not come true, you have more strength than you realize, and the world has more people who care about you than you know or could ever know.

5. Loneliness

A research paper that summarized findings from 35 studies involving over 75,000 people reported that perceived loneliness increased mortality by 22 percent.[11]

I recognize my need to belong, which is a universal human feeling.[12] However, as much as I love people, I know relationships are nuanced. Even the kindest of people might act ornery on their difficult days. Sometimes, even the closest colleagues are so lost in thoughts that they would rather ignore me in the elevator. So, accept the day-to-day relationship undulations and do not let them create turbulence in your mind.

You may disagree with me, but I have found one of the best ways to curb loneliness is to decrease my need for others' presence, attention, or adulation to feel good about myself. Giving others the freedom to leave works well to bring them closer to you. Further, with the decreased need, your presence becomes more authentic and freer of any personal agenda, providing you with uplifting feelings from the tiniest of encounters. Finding joy through tiny informal encounters all day long with different people creates what researchers call "relational diversity." Research shows people's relational diversity, measured as having a broad "social portfolio" through which you can find positivity, is an excellent predictor of well-being.[13]

In addition to a positive connection with the self and sprinkling uplifting micro-connections, the simplest way to decrease the need for others' adulations is to embrace a charitable purpose. Research convincingly shows that people with a vital purpose guiding their lives are much less likely to feel lonely.[14]

I remember a story I heard as a child about an old lady who worked on a farm. She would spend days in the fields with the crops, having no connection with another human being. When asked by a local if she ever felt lonely, she looked surprised. "I didn't even think about it. I have no time to feel lonely!" She was totally in flow in the company of her closest friends — the crops.

A moment that brings Richa into flow is cooking. When people ask me for restaurant recommendations, I often say my home is the best one in town. Once while watching her cook, I was thinking about the relationship between oil and water. They may sit together for a long time but don't mix. You need an emulsifier to bring them together. That emulsifier in our life is finding commonalities.

Given how much the world is obsessed these days with reminding us about our differences, it is important we counter that by focusing on our similarities with each other. As long as we consider others different and get spooked by our differences, we will stay separate. The moment we ponder over our common backgrounds, shared dreams, overlapping fears, similar passions, and united motivations, our one plus one will become eleven.

The two motivations

Sustaining behavior change (to say no to life limiters) needs time and energy. Investing time and energy needs motivation, both internal and external. This is a common topic of conversation, so I will summarize a few ideas here.

Your internal motivation comes from your passion to leave the world a little better than you found. For instance, I am committed to helping create a kinder, more hopeful, and happier world for our planet's children. Humbly, I feel I am helpful to others, a pursuit I strive to expand and deepen. I have also spent several decades learning about resilience, happiness, well-being, relationships, parenting, and burnout mitigation concepts. I want to synthesize and share that knowledge with others, which I can only do if I stay healthy. All of this drives my internal motivation.

Helpful comparisons drive my external motivation. They can be upward or downward. My upward comparison is with someone very close to me — my ninety-year-old father, Sahib. Sahib walks several miles a day, is very actively engaged with learning world's current affairs, eats well, and loves to show his culinary finesse once in a while. Compared to his loved ones, classmates, and co-workers, he has beaten all the health and survival odds. Part of it might be his resilient genes, but a considerable part is his lifestyle, which is simple, active, and peace-loving. Like him, I want to be present in my children's lives, to the extent they want! This thought motivates me to take better care of myself.

As a physician, I have seen countless patients who did not take good care of their bodies and, as a result, spent several decades in and out of the hospital, much more than desired. Sometimes, I use their experience as a downward comparison, though that seldom helps me sustain a behavior change for a long time.

In addition, empower one or more people to be your accountability buddy. Richa, Gauri, and Sia all nag me to get off the couch, always successfully.

Talking about motivation reminds me of a patient I met a few years ago. She had been smoking for more than fifty years. We had tried everything under the sun, but it didn't work.

One day, she quit cold turkey, and for good. I asked her how that happened. She said, "I leaned forward to kiss my grandson. He took two steps back and said, Grandma, you stink. That was it." No wonder the word emotion has motion in it — it moves you.

I learned three things from this story. One, strong emotional motivations can drive an immediate and enduring change. Two, we need people who can tell us the truth. Third, if we have the strength to look at the truth in its face and act on it, we might experience many transformative moments in our life.

One final detail: You can turn your story of failure into a story of success by sharing with others. As director of well-being at a medical school, I started a program called "My story." Prominent staff and faculty talked to the students about their failures and answered any questions. It became the most well-attended program and continues to help students, now almost a decade later. So, don't be shy in sharing your stories if they can help others. Perhaps you are successful today because someone was courageous and kind to share their story with you.

We carry a multitude of contradictory impulses within us — for selfishness, greed, ego, anger, impulsiveness, envy, and malice, and for generosity, gratitude, humility, peace, patience, collegiality, and forgiveness. These contradictory impulses guide us to loathe ourselves at one moment and love at another. Where do they come from and how do we integrate them to create harmony?

Through the previous four sections I have been itching to share the two-part model of self that I use to understand the bag of contradictions that is me. Our further foray into self-love will entail negotiating a bit more challenging terrain that will need you to open your heart to yourself even more. We are walking into the world of self-compassion, self-acceptance, and self-forgiveness. Let's rediscover the self so we learn how to be more effortless in embodying a compassionate, accepting, and forgiving disposition toward ourselves.

Your "Self": A Model

18

Self, An Introduction

---— ✤✤✤ ———

> The priceless can't be measured in any currency. Think of all you have that money can't buy. It will tell you your true worth.

August 27th, 2124. Your holographic self is in a virtual-reality office for a follow-up on your "self-scan." "Amazing progress," Ida, your health-span coach, beams. "Your courage areas show strong activity, the self-confidence network is expanding, and that dark shadow of self-rejection is barely visible now. How do you feel?"

"Stronger every day," you say, matching up with Ida's energy. "In the summary report, though, I saw some mention about fear."

"Yes, I was coming to that. That red enhancement on the left shows you still have dense old hubs of unresolved fears. They correlate with your inflammatory gene activity."

Ida designs a personal "dismantle-my-fears" program for you. A follow up scan will be in three months.

Wouldn't it be nice if we could look at our self in colors? We would no longer need to convince people that our feelings are real. Unfortunately, we aren't there yet.

Let's go as far as the current science can take us, and a little bit beyond, to understand our self. Science presently hasn't figured out how to study the non-material realm. Further, science is one way to study the world, not the only way. Science assumes a rational basis for how the world operates that we can understand and then influence it for our benefit. So, we will keep a rational underpinning for every step we take past the scientific realm. Let's start with a thought experiment that has tickled the imagination of countless thinkers.

Ship of Theseus

A mythical king, Theseus, founder of Athens, rescued Athenian children from King Minos and then escaped on a ship to Delos. His feat was celebrated every year by taking the ship on a pilgrimage. Over time, the ship's old planks decayed and were replaced until every single plank was new. With all the planks now different than the original, would this ship have the same or a distinct identity? In other words, is the ship defined by its planks, how they function together, or something else? Your response, both yes and no, although in conflict, is defensible.

Let's draw a parallel between this parable and the human body. If a human being starts getting organ transplants, at what point, if any, would that person cease to be them? We know that a heart or a face transplant doesn't change a person's identity. What about a brain transplant, if that becomes a possibility in the future?

In other words, is there a "self" within us that transcends our physical being?

You might not need to answer this question if you lived in complete solitude on the far side of the moon with no "other." But we live in a social world within a language construct where I, me, and mine are some of the more commonly used words. So, who are we referring to when we say I?

Defining self

Self is the essence that separates us from every other entity. We develop this identity by integrating inputs from two sources:

the intrapersonal (the inner environment), and
the interpersonal (the outside world).

Both the intrapersonal and the interpersonal are perceived in two different ways:

instinctive, and
intentional.

A young child has limited intentional capacity, so she is vulnerable to the littlest negative feedback. However, as we get older, our maturing executive cortex helps us be intentional about blending both the positive and negative inputs to create a balanced perspective that helps us grow.

Simultaneous with developing intentionality, we evolve a self that gives us a central place of presence from which we observe and experience the world.

Contemplatives, scientists, and philosophers have each taken a novel and sometimes opposite stance on the self. For some, the self is all there is. Others deny the self, assuming it is as tangible as the center of gravity. A few, particularly neuroscientists, think of self as a perception, our sixth sense if you will, that emerges from neural activity in specific brain regions. Let's hear from neuroscientists first before turning to the contemplatives.

Neural self

Neurologically, does the self emerge from the brain's activity, or is the self a distinct entity that plays on the brain? Over the years, researchers have correlated perceiving the self with activity in several brain areas.

One of these areas is the posterior cingulate cortex (PCC). A team of researchers led by Dr. Judson Brewer, whom I hosted for a keynote about a decade ago, found that self-reference components correlate with PCC activity.[1] They point out that meditators who transcend the self into a state of "effortless doing" can quiet their PCC.[2] Very interestingly, similar brain areas show deactivation in people receiving psychedelics who also report transcending the self.[3-4]

An area that predictably activates with self-identity is the medial prefrontal cortex (mPFC).[5] Our brain's mPFC is involved in self-awareness and self-enhancement and is thus closely associated with social functioning.

Your awareness of your physical body, particularly its internal visceral state, is sensed by the insula, a brain area tucked deep inside the cortex between the frontal and temporal lobes.[6]

Memory brain systems are also important for constructing the self. From the memory perspective, the self combines both personal autobiographical memories (recollection of episodes from your life)[7] and a memory of the context and general knowledge of the world.[8] In fact, your sense of self and memory are so deeply integrated that some scientists call them the self-memory system.

Despite all the advances, our neuroscientific understanding of the self is still early. Where do all our thoughts, emotions, memories, perceptions, and values converge? Does our brain's orchestra have a master conductor, is it a matrix with many masters that take turns, or something else? Neuroscientists presently don't have a definitive answer.[9]

This makes me ask, "Am I just a clump of DNA wandering around like driftwood, or is my reality that of an inner pure essence enveloped by a physical shell on an intentional journey?" I have concepts that work for me, which I will continue to share through this book and beyond. My current responses, however, are only placeholders that the next generation, with better technology and greater wisdom, will and must edit.

Donald Winnicott, a twentieth-century English pediatrician and psychoanalyst, wisely stated, "A word like self...knows more than we do." So, let's stay humble in our assertions as we forge ahead to understand the self, ever expanding our imaginations beyond what our sensory system and the present state of science can show us.[10]

Please rest assured that we aren't taking a metaphysical exit that will culminate in a secret levitation mantra. We strive to give words to our daily experience of our relationship with ourselves.

Without a scientifically reproducible scan and a conclusively proven neural structure that hosts the self, we need to develop a model, if only as a placeholder, that can help us decipher our struggles and pave a path for thriving. How do we develop that model — build or break? Let's pursue that next.

19
Build or Break?

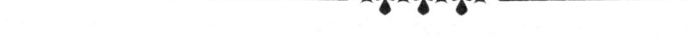

> A truly spiritual idea unites us instead of dividing us.

Broadly, most scientific disciplines take two approaches to learning about an entity: build or break. Building entails adding the parts to construct the whole. Breaking involves splitting the whole into its parts.

Splitting is the commoner approach to studying natural entities since they have already been built for us. For instance, in botany, we study a flower by learning its parts: sepals, petals, stamens, and carpels. Similarly, we learn about the human body by studying its different organs, and we study organs, such as the brain, by looking at their parts.

No matter their disagreement, most scientists, philosophers, and contemplatives agree about one detail — we can't build our "self" *de novo*. It is nature's gift to us. So, deconstruction might be the right approach to learning about the self.

You'll notice that this approach, i.e. understanding an entity or a concept by looking at its constituents, is a recurring theme in most disciplines. Self is perhaps the most complex entity to deconstruct. So, please bear with me if I occasionally make assumptions based more on common sense than published research in the interest of simplicity.

My first fling with my self happened almost four decades ago amidst a difficult life phase as a fifteen-year-old. Let's travel back to a rural, state-funded school in North Central India.

Pure water

My daughters tell me that I totally missed out on fun in my school years. I agree. I was a boringly idealistic middle schooler who seldom spoke curse words, didn't hang out with the "cool kids," and never played pranks on my teachers. As an uncool kid whose growth spurt got delayed because of a neurological condition, I was a natural target for bullies. On top of that, the medicines used to treat my condition left me drowsy and dizzy, affecting my learning.

All of that hurt my self-worth, before I knew what that word meant. But I was lucky, because my English teacher, Mr. Kamesh, believed in me. I could say anything to him without feeling judged.

One morning, during a particularly rough week, he called me to his office to share an insight about water. I had no idea his thoughts would stay with me for the rest of my life, and in some ways, change my life's trajectory. Here is an approximate sequence of what I recall about my discussion that day.

Mr. Kamesh kept a glass half filled with water on the table.

"What do you see here?" he asked.

"A glass of water?" I was confused about where he was going.

"Yes, that's right. Dirty or clean?"

"Clean, I think," I said after peering through the glass.

Next, he took out a plastic bag full of dirt and emptied a few spoons in the water. After stirring gently, he asked, "What do you see now?"

"Dirty water," I said.

He nodded. "What might happen if we leave this water still for a few days?"

"The dust will settle at the bottom."

"Leaving the pure water at the top," his eyes brightened. "What do you learn from this?"

"If you leave the water still, it gets pure." I wasn't sure if I got the right answer or at least the one he wanted.

"Yes, that's good. But here is an even more important lesson. Behind every collection of dirty water is pure water that you can reclaim. Mud starts with pure water, and in the end, the same pure water will separate to leave the dirt. Mud has both dirt and water. While the dirt is more visible, the water keeps it together; otherwise, the wind will blow it away."

It was all common sense to me thus far. I didn't know what to do with this information. That's when Mr. Kamesh connected it with my life.

"I know you are going through tough times. Remember that your life's challenges — losing the soccer game, being called names, bad grades, your diagnosis — are all the dirt. You are the pure and priceless water that the dirt can't touch. You have a choice. You can assume you are the dirt or consider yourself the water. Which one do you choose?"

"The water," I said.

Mr. Kamesh looked happy with my choice. "Think about it and let me know if you have any questions. You are a good boy. I am proud of you."

As I walked out of his office, I wasn't sure if I got the entire message. But as the months rolled by and I got to talk to Mr. Kamesh a bit more, the fog lifted.

"In every clump of mud is pure water. It starts with water and ends with water, but somehow, dirt takes over in the middle. The more I can identify with the water instead of the dirt, the more power I will have over my struggles."

In its simplest way, this metaphor invited me to focus on the positives in my life. Yes, I had a neurological condition, but I had access to treatment. Some boys called me names, but many others were kind.

As I moved toward high school and then college, I was partially successful at holding on to Mr. Kamesh's teachings that the real me, my essence, my self, remains unblemished by anything that happens to my physical body or mind. This latter realization became a firm conviction as my brain's pre-frontal cortex matured.

Over the years, my thinking changed in two specific ways.

One, remembering that I was the pure essence helped me persevere despite my illness and the challenge of assimilating the medical school curriculum while having to take a sedative medicine. It helped me stay hopeful. Through failures and disappointments, I always believed if I worked hard and had a pure heart, it would all work out in the end. That belief helped me hold myself to higher values.

Two, when I met people, I started thinking about the innocence and purity everyone carried, even though their annoying mind may have made it invisible to others and themselves. This realization took much longer to influence my daily experience.

My neuroscience education gave me a better vocabulary by teaching me about the higher cortical and lower limbic brains. Dabbling in meditation gave me a new perspective, this time in the language of changing and changeless.

Changing and changeless

I sometimes travel forward from my birth to the present moment in my meditations. In those trips, once the outer turbulence quiets, I sense the still background behind my thoughts and emotions. That part of me has stayed constant, walking along with the rest that continues to change.

While the superficial turbulence feels slightly different each day, the spacious stillness remains changeless. Which one is me — the turbulence, the stillness, or both? I believe both, as the figure below shows (Figure 5). Just as the stage and the actors merge to create the experience, so do the changing and changeless part of me.

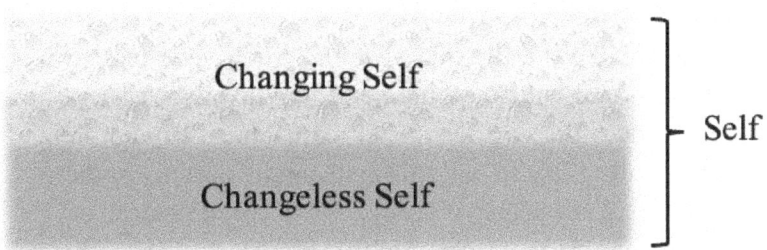

Figure 5. The two-part self: Changing and Changeless

I invite you to pause and think about what within you has been changing from your birth and what is changeless. Together, they merge to create you, your self.

One more detail — you can imagine the changing and changeless blended together like a smoothie, or you can imagine them as two separate coexisting mutually supportive entities, like a two-flower bouquet. I don't have a definitive answer, but one day while clipping my nails I had an interesting chain of thoughts that tremendously helped my understanding. It didn't solve the smoothie dilemma, but it provided me insights into what is in the blender. Let's visit that moment.

Spiritual nails

After I carefully pared my human talons, I looked at the curvilinear trimmings before discarding them. I felt no connection to the little fragments, zero emotions. But just a few minutes prior, they were a part of my physical body. Many of my fellow humans spend top dollar to decorate these pincers.

I carried this thought forward and imagined if I lost a body part, such as my little toe. I would remain the same person. Opposite to losing, receiving someone else's body part also won't change my self. A cherished colleague of mine has received a heart transplant. With someone else's heart in her body, she is still the same person she was before the transplant.

All of this led me to a simple conclusion: Our core identity transcends our physical body. Illness, aging, or other physical circumstances do not change it. Similarly, our brain states — asleep or awake — do not affect it. You stay the same person, through different sleep stages and during anesthesia.

Presently, like the far side of a black hole, this part of us hasn't been photographed and isn't measurable by any available scientific instrument. We experience the world in an expanding circumference from this changeless core. I like to call this unchanging part of us, the essence of life, or in short, Esse (Esse means being, our essential nature).

I also recognize another part of the self that evolves with changing neural activity. Activate the brain's reward network, and it becomes happy; tickle the amygdala, and it experiences fear; stir the pain matrix, and it experiences hurt. It goes in the background when the brain sleeps and is online first thing in the morning. It is essential to life's expression, but it can also be a nuisance. I call it my Psyche (the totality of our mind — conscious, subconscious, and unconscious).

Esse and Psyche together create the self. As I stated, this doesn't solve the smoothie problem. Nevertheless, parsing the self will greatly improve our access to self-love, particularly for those who find it difficult to embrace or fully grasp self-compassion, self-acceptance, and self-forgiveness.

Who knew clipping nails could be such an illuminating experience!

The totality of our world is divided into two units: the experienced (the external world) and the experiencer (the self). We experience the inanimate and the world's living beings through the physical body, the mind, and our deeper essence (Figure 6).

| Inanimate |
| Living beings |
| Physical Body |
| Psyche/Mind |
| Deeper Essence |

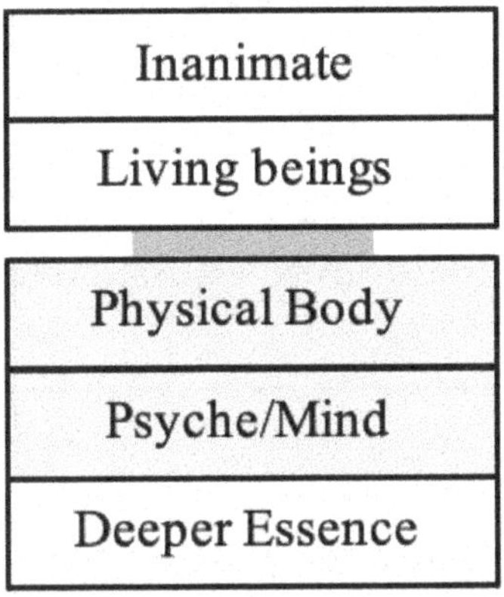

Figure 6. The totality

Based on what I shared above, you could consider your physical body as both the experiencer and the experienced. Some traditions treat the mind the same as the physical body (i.e., both the experiencer and the experienced). That's an intriguing way of looking at the self, helping us soften our relationship with our thoughts.

For now, I feel comfortable considering our mind (Psyche) and our essence deeper than the mind (Esse) as the two elements constituting our experiencer (our self).

Next, I invite you to pause for a moment and discern what I have shared so far in the context of your beliefs.

20
What Do You Think?

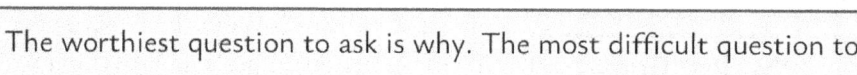

> The worthiest question to ask is why. The most difficult question to answer is why.

At this point, which one of the following positions would you take?

1. I am not sure if the two-part model (Self = Esse + Psyche) is right or wrong, but I am willing to work with it.

2. I am not sure if the two-part model is right or wrong, but I am <u>not</u> willing to work with it.

3. The two-part model is wrong, and I am unwilling to work with it.

4. The two-part model is wrong, but I am willing to work with it.

5. The two-part model is right, and I am willing to work with it.

6. The two-part model is right, but I am unwilling to work with it.

We could add a few more choices but I invite you to pick one from the above before proceeding.

Biostatistician George E.P. Box astutely stated in a 1978 publication, "All models are wrong but some are useful." Scientific models last until a better model that can more fully explain the newer observations supersedes them. Since 1969, when we landed on the moon, numerous physics and math models have come and gone. Nevertheless, our understanding and computing power at that time (which I am told was equal to what you have in your present Smartphone) was enough to send three people 239,000 miles away and bring them back safely.[1]

As science develops, the suggested Esse/Psyche approach will be deemed too simplistic and superseded by a more evidence-based model. Nevertheless, I strongly feel that it serves as a good placeholder to help us move from self-rejection to self-love. Toward that end, I'll be immensely grateful if you are willing to work with it, at least for the time we are together. You are welcome to use different names, if you wish, based on your background and belief systems.

You might be intrigued that in my journey, I have encountered a few contemplatives who stated they have tangibly experienced and seen their Esse. Remarkably, their individual descriptions were nearly identical even though they didn't know each other or what the other person said. But it is a private experience that isn't easily replicable for most of us. So, I won't dabble in it further, at least not in this book.

We could debate subjectivity versus objectivity for a very long time and not reach anywhere. Instead, let me talk to you about how I arrived at some clarity after hearing about Mike's missed stop sign.

Missed stop sign

I met Mike, a forty-five-year-old software programmer, for a stress management consult a few years ago. I saw pain in his eyes. Halfway into our appointment, he opened up and shared a life-altering event.

Mike was driving back home late at night. In a moment of drowsy distraction, he missed the stop sign and was T boned by a truck coming from the left side. A few days later he had to bury his two-year-old son who was in the car seat. "I feel ashamed for what I did. I can never forgive myself," Mike said between his sobs. He had tried all the different conventional therapies and medications to no avail. How would you comfort Mike if you were me?

I shared with Mike the limitations of the human brain. His tired, sleep-deprived brain caused his eyes to involuntarily shut at the wrong moment. We discussed the difference between shame and guilt and that the guilt will never go away. We also discussed how unchecked shame could keep his mind riled up for decades, exacting an enormous cost on him and his family.

I could see him ever so slightly shift toward feeling validated for his pain, recognizing that although he was negligent, he wasn't intentional. Yet, Mike was struggling with having two conflicting thoughts at the same time. How could he honor his son's memory while at the same time move forward and find peace? Feeling peaceful seemed disrespectful.

I invited him to consider that notwithstanding the mishap and the guilt, he still had a preserved core of purity (his Esse). Despite something very bad happening at his hands unintentionally, his other two kids, wife, and older parents needed him, and he wasn't there. They needed not just his physical presence but for him to feel worthy again.

Love shines the brightest in the hearts purified by wisdom borne of suffering. With time and effort, from a place of Esse within him, Mike could "see" his suffering instead of fusing with it. He could see his benign intentions, and although he couldn't progress to self-forgiveness, he could find self-compassion.

Self-compassion started him on a journey to again be a good dad, a devoted husband, a loving son, and an effective professional. Without it, he had given up on life.

Good people, bad situations

Much of my work involves meeting good people caught in difficult situations. Situations like health care professionals whose errors led to catastrophic outcomes, workers whose misjudgments led to avoidable accidents, executives whose lives got destroyed by a single financial mistake, and professors whose carelessness got them into a plagiarism scandal. Every single day you can walk with your head held high is a phenomenal day.

At the other extreme, people are affected by illegal, immoral, or negligent behaviors of their colleagues, friends, loved ones, or random strangers. A very successful and educated colleague found her husband of twenty years philandering. She felt ashamed because of it. The reason? When confronted with the evidence, her husband retorted, "It's all your fault. You pushed me away to someone else." Really?

In all these instances, accessing a safe, calm place within helps people shift from incessant thoughts of self-judgment to a healing presence. Touching that space, even for a brief moment, silences their "inner bully," helping them get unstuck and start moving forward while honoring their past. In other words, they shift from shame to guilt to self-worth and eventually to self-love.

Countless people struggling with their unruly or overwhelmed mind need help today. They want to transcend their inner loneliness by embracing self-worth and self-love. But they don't know how. The belief and access to a pure innocent Esse within them can provide healing to many who have experienced life's worst traumas, have begun to hate their physical body, and can't quickly reframe because their mind is fused with the trauma.

Patients with a disfiguring physical illness might find peace when they connect with their inner unseen beauty. They don't have to create that beauty; just reclaim what is already there. People with self-rejection can find self-love when they believe that deep down, they are unblemished.

Let's conclude this chapter by revisiting neuroscience where we have been trying to understand the brain by looking at its individual parts. I will share an experience using my favorite topic — donuts!

Brain eyeing a donut

Imagine your brain looking at a donut. The brain's reward network thinks, "I want this donut to be part of my body because the caloric gain will come in handy fighting the next Neanderthal, which can happen any minute." The fear network thinks about all the unhealthy calories, cholesterol, sugar, and salt in the donut. The prefrontal cortex, the rational part of the brain, thinks that although unhealthy, an occasional donut is fine.

Your decision integrates these three inputs and depends on which brain area predominates. If you are starving, the reward network might carry the show, but if you just found out that your blood sugar is inching higher, the fear network might overrule every other part.

One final aspect is that despite the different brain areas evaluating the donut, you do not say, "Let me consider what my left amygdala is saying!"

Instead, you merge all these inputs and experience the donut with the entire brain.

If you travel to the time of Aristotle when they believed that the brain served as the cooling agent for the heart, you will have no idea of its different parts. Any model of the brain having seventeen individual major structures, and eighty-six billion neurons would have been absurd. I wonder if, at some future point, the same might be true about our self. Could our scientific instruments advance one day to measure what seems immeasurable right now?

Just as we can measure heart rate variability to get feedback about our relaxation, it would be nice to know we are indeed progressing in compassion or mastering our fears. I wonder what would happen if a potential criminal could see their pure Esse in real time. Despite their Psyche misguiding them, seeing their pure Esse would be a powerful influence on them to mend their ways.

The fantasy of today becomes the science of tomorrow. I invite you to consider that every human has a precious, pure essence within them.[2] To me, it offers an egalitarian, hopeful way of looking at humanity. It also affirms our ability to treat ourselves with compassion, acceptance, and forgiveness, three flavors of love that are a perfect antidote to inner loneliness.

You can stay with Esse or choose any other name you like, including your chosen religious figure. Further, consider connecting with others' Esse in your daily interactions, starting with close friends and loved ones.

Your belief that every person has an invisible purity within them, more than any scientific construct or therapy, can help you with compassion, acceptance, and forgiveness of others and self. It took away my social anxiety, replacing it with a non-judgmental healing presence.

A healing presence is desperately needed today in our personal lives and the business world, as we continue testing the limits of our capitalistic experiment that is cannibalizing our positive emotions and connections and giving birth to all kinds of greed, fear, and rage. Fortunately, we have already started moving in that direction using different verbiage, such as emotional intelligence, conscious capitalism, servant leadership, socially responsible business, and others. We must accelerate our collective evolution, which moves our presence from instinctive to intentional, fabricated to authentic, and evaluative to healing. That's where we are headed next — our presence.

21
Your Presence

---❖❖❖---

> Best not to multitask in relationships. Partial presence feels worse than absence.

It took me over ten years of training before I saw my first patient as a "real doctor" without anyone supervising me. This is common for physicians. The reason is simple. While you can memorize the causes, consequences, and treatment of illnesses, the finesse to effortlessly bring it all together in a high-stake, high-speed environment when you may not have much time to think takes lots of experience.

The same applies to the quality of your presence. While you may embody your best behavior for two hours at dinner, it takes time and effort to make enduring changes where you embody a healing presence all day long every day. Your progress occurs in three overlapping steps.

Step 1. Evaluative presence

In this state, you make rapid judgments, which research shows can happen in less than 100 milliseconds.[1-2] Our judgments have two opposite goals: seeking and averting, aligned with the primal biological goal of eating, not getting eaten, and reproducing.

We seek experiences that activate our brain's reward network and avert experiences that activate the pain matrix or amygdala. In this state, you are constantly comparing and judging, competing to trounce your rivals, and living in a polarized world.

An evaluative disposition was helpful for our physically threatened ancestors. But an evaluative overdrive amidst predominantly emotional threats is an antithesis of contentment, compassion, altruism, and peace. I promise you, most people you find annoying in your life home in this state.

Step 2. Observing presence

As we grow, we learn the art of increasing the space between attention and interpretation. The length of this precious space, to a limit, directly correlates with your patience and thoughtfulness. You start recognizing that your rapid judgments are fatiguing and often misinformed. You step back and become a better observer of the truth.

A useful byproduct is greater joy. You start finding ordinary daisies gorgeous. Food tastes better. You feel grateful for a stranger's smile, spot new designs in cloud formations, and don't get bored doing simple chores such as folding laundry and loading the dishwasher. You are now mindful and ready to move further to a more profound presence.

Step 3. Healing presence

A mindful presence is but a passing phase to take you home to where you embody a healing disposition, first only occasionally and eventually throughout the day. It doesn't matter where you are or what you do. You could send silent compassion while ordering your coffee, booking a flight, talking to a teller, or negotiating with your teenager. Gradually, from occasionally visiting Planet Kindness, you make it your home.

In your daily interactions, you remember that people fear becoming inconsequential and being forgotten. You help them feel they will always matter and be remembered.

Simultaneously, the world notices your healing presence. People find you calm. They comment on how they feel centered when they are with you. As you advance, your struggles with your mind fade. Greed, ego, and fear seldom touch you. You become much more effective at your work. The essence of life in you, your Esse, starts shining through.

Imagine a world where we all embody a healing presence all the time. We all radiate the persona of a sage — eight billion sages walking on the planet. I believe this will happen sometime in the future. I want to be there when that happens!

Being a sage doesn't mean you wear saffron clothes after taking a vow of celibacy. It means together, we create a world where trust and respect are the default options, where I love your children as much as you do, and vice versa. Won't that be nice?

Two questions

Back to the real world! I ask you two questions. Please pause and think deeply since the responses to these questions have deeply influenced my every relationship. Answer them with your best guess based on the preponderance of your beliefs.

Q1. The <u>likely</u> nature of your Esse is –
a. Innocent, pure, and sacred
b. Scheming, impure, and mundane

Q2. Esse is present –
a. In only a select few
b. In every human being

Here are my responses to the two questions.

A1: My Esse is innocent, pure, and sacred (a)
In my last forty years of meeting monks and contemplative masters, I have been fortunate to meet a few people who, with complete conviction, "know" that the correct answer is a. Their conviction and commitment to living a life of altruism have helped my journey tremendously.

Think about when you may have experienced a presence where all your concerns, desires, and hurts disappeared. It could be while rocking a sleeping six-month-old, playing with a puppy, or listening to your grandma. During these moments, the peace and joy you experience from touching your innocence and purity is the nature of your Esse.

I feel worthy, hopeful, and empowered, knowing that having my compassionate, accepting, loving, and forgiving Esse within me gives me everything I need to heal myself.

A2: Esse is present in every human being (b)
"All humans are created equal" is the spirit of the constitution. In humanity's brutal past, most of us, including Aristotle and Socrates, didn't believe in equality. Keeping slaves was the norm. The same brain that today willingly agrees to donate its body's kidney to a stranger was willingly raising

arms against toddlers. Sadly, we continue to be a work in progress since our brain's compassion highways are still under construction.

The belief that we all have a pure essence within us will accelerate our progress toward an egalitarian world. It is one of the most powerful, if not the most powerful, beliefs that has changed my relationship with fellow humans.

Feeling inferior or superior are weak and vulnerable states; feeling equal is genuinely empowering. Once you believe that every person has a priceless Esse, then when it comes to respecting people, it matters little to you whether one gets by on food stamps or is a multimillionaire. Every person deserves your respect just because they are human. Even the thought of abusing someone or taking advantage of the vulnerable would not come to you.

Carrying this belief has improved my self-worth, enriched every relationship, and healed old wounds. It has taken away my social anxiety while infusing empowering humility. I find it easier to experience uplifting, nurturing, and high-quality moments with others, while at the same time feel peaceful in my own company.

You can expand this thought to animals, but let's save that for another time. I do believe, though, that my canine son, Simba, has a purer than pure Esse!

Here is what bothers me. If we all have a pure Esse within us, why has our world seen tyrants who have treated fellow humans worse than objects? Why do the top 1 percent hoard as much wealth as the bottom 90% combined, forcing over seven hundred million people on our planet to live on less than $2.15 per day? Why did many privileged Titanic passengers traveling in the first class not extend a helping hand to ones in the third class? It is because our Esse stays silent, hidden in the layers of complexity weaved by a part of us that is still a work in progress — our Psyche.

22
Our Complex Psyche

> Seeing the good in the bad isn't denying the bad. It is denying the bad from taking over your mind.

A short drive from my home is the mighty Mississippi River. Over the years, I have seen different colors and moods of the river — calm, playful, energized, angry, and more. The river's countenance sometimes changes by the hour, depending on the rain, wind, and other factors.

Like every other river, the Mississippi is mysterious. Even if I get a Ph.D. on the "life of the Mississippi," I could never claim to fully know her. She has a hidden past and an unknown future; her physical being might look calm in La Crosse, WI, but a few hours' drive away, she could be courting rafters up for the challenge.

Our Psyche is not too dissimilar. It is complex and ever-changing. In my talks, I often show the brain video of a neuroscience colleague while he was relaxing in the fMRI machine, letting his mind wander. At each moment, his brain showed a slightly different activity pattern, very much like a flowing river.

Psyche defined

With that background, here is a working definition of Psyche: *an ever-changing construct created by a constant stream of thoughts and emotions.* This construct has many elements: your instincts, attention, memories (conscious and repressed), intellect, thoughts, executive functions, learnings, feelings, and language.

Imagine placing a mirror in New York's Times Square. Thousands of people will pass by your mirror every day. But at any one moment, this mirror reflects only the person whose face is in front of it. Your Psyche is similar, constantly reflecting the present-moment experience.

Many external factors influence your thoughts and emotions. Your perceived professional success, financial status, physical appearance, respect from others, thoughts about the future, and more. Your set of twenty thousand genes, the brain's networking, early childhood experiences, personality, expectations from the self, and learnings over the years also affect your thinking train. All these converge to create your brain's present state that generates your thoughts, feelings, and behaviors.

Perceived

Watch the word perceived in the previous paragraph. Your evaluation of the present moment has very little to do with reality. A good friend of mine, whose work may have saved up to one hundred million lives (I'm not exaggerating), struggles with low self-worth.

"Post-achievement depression" is common among the super successful. Researchers call it the Arrival fallacy, the illusion that goal achievement will lead to lasting happiness.[1] For instance, in a classic study, researchers found that professors who had received tenure in the previous five years were no happier than those who didn't get tenure. However, assistant professors looking for tenures consistently overestimated the joy they would experience in the future with this accomplishment.[2]

The dissatisfaction and lack of happiness after achievements (that we thought would make us happy) is particularly painful. Before achievement we at least carried a hope, albeit a false one, that success would make us happier; now even that hope is lost.

Powering our discontent is the sad reality that many of us give others the power to influence our perception of the self, irrespective of whether they care about us. We take their negative feedback literally, not realizing that their words might be coming from a place of envy. Further, negative and more recent evaluations in our math outweigh the positive and remote ones. That's how someone with a million likes on social media might lose their cool when one person at a restaurant acts rude toward them.

This process of relinquishing power starts very early in childhood, just when our neurons start their selective pruning and are busy deciding who they will buddy up with for the foreseeable future. In children, others' evaluation sets the tone for self-evaluation. Children thus create a life script, a GPS for their journey, that does not necessarily take them through the most scenic highways toward a happy destination.

Many children hear words that could create permanent scars in their developing brain, given that two out of three children in the U.S. have experienced adverse childhood experiences (ACE).[3]

Even in the absence of an obvious ACE from an adult, our Psyche can get easily injured by derogatory comments from people our age, particularly if they attack our physical appearance. As I shared with you earlier, that happened to me when I was barely ten.

My countenance

My Psyche got a big blow when my first crush rejected me outright based on my physical appearance. It took me two decades to recover from that affront. Even now, I sometimes look at my profile disapprovingly!

Over the years, I have talked to so many young people who lost their passion for life because of one or two cruel comments about their appearance or another attribute. Such comments, by dismantling children's early efforts at developing a positive, nurturing connection with oneself, can leave a long-lasting impact when the brain networks aren't fully mature.

As we get older, we evolve, hopefully moving from evaluative to observer self. With this evolution, what matters at a young age no longer bothers us.

For instance, as a young child, I cared a lot about pressing the elevator buttons; as a teenager, my hairstyle defined my day; as a new researcher, my publications mattered a lot. But now all of this seems so trivial. Let me know if you still care about pressing the elevator buttons. If yes, then we need to talk!

Unseen shadows

One of the few times I got very upset with Richa was when she called me careless for misplacing the car keys. She was factually right, but her words hit a sensitive nerve. Later, as I thought about my disproportionate response, I realized that it had to do with unpleasant childhood memories of being called clumsy and inept.

Many of us carry shadows of previous unprocessed trauma. Most children experience fear, anger, guilt, shame, sadness, worry, and disgust at some point. Unfortunately, many also experience neglect, abandonment, and abuse. Children experience these scourges at a time when they do not know how to process their negative emotions. As a result, they repress these painful feelings and, unable to separate themselves from these feelings, begin rejecting themselves.

Your unexpectedly strong reaction to an accusation shows an underlying predisposition that you repressed and rejected. Walking upstream on your feelings, sometimes with the help of a coach, might help you uncover a painful past. Awareness starts your process of healing. Since you can't go back and change the past, the best approach now is to cultivate greater self-compassion, self-acceptance, and self-forgiveness.

Friend, I do not know you personally, and perhaps you do not know me very well. But, likely, we carry similar past shadows lodged in our Psyche. I know how it feels, so as I continue the work to free myself of these shadows, I want to reassure you that it gets better with time, as you develop a more secure relationship with yourself.

Could we keep it simpler?

I love simplicity. So, I owe you a little more explanation of why imagining ourselves as a combination of Esse and Psyche can help.

I have met the kindest, most well-meaning corporate executives who couldn't resist back-dating options when the opportunity presented itself. Almost every single man I have asked has either philandered or fantasized about that possibility. Many good people wonder how nice it might be if their supervisor mysteriously disappeared over the weekend. Despite working hard to live by timeless values, very likely, if I face extreme persecution or massive disparity, I will revolt.

Further, despite working on myself for over three decades, I still sometimes am visited by thoughts I wouldn't be proud to own. In meeting the self and others, I have a choice: assume that my messed-up mind is all I have, or consider that behind the muddiest puddle, once you separate the dirt, you have crystal clear pure water. Many years ago, I decided to choose the latter, and that choice has been transformative.

Parsing Esse from Psyche has given me easier access to my purity despite my many imperfections. Without such distinction, my negativity bias effortlessly pulled my attention to the hurtful and guilt-worthy, like a magnet pulls iron beads.

Limiting the hurtful to only a small part of me, not the whole of me, and being able to "look" at the dimly lit corners of my Psyche with healing eyes has helped me make better decisions and preserved my sanity so I do not let adversity become a catastrophe.

The earlier you can contain the fire, the better. Most large forest fires start as small unnoticed bushfires that didn't get contained. The same is true for global wars that have killed and maimed hundreds of millions of people. So, I invite you to preemptively think and practice identifying with Esse in yourself and others. That will help you preserve grace during difficult moments, transforming them into blissful memories.

Giving Grace

Simon was the town sheriff in a city of about ten thousand. He invited my team to share our resilience program with all his staff. As someone who walked the walk, he implemented resilience practices in his personal life. One of the practices was a commitment to kindness through assuming positive intent in others.

A few months after our course, he was playing baseball with his buddies. One of the foul balls went into a neighbor's yard. When Simon went to retrieve it, the neighbor refused. "What if the ball hit someone in my home?" the neighbor yelled.

Simon had an urge to jump the fence and snatch the ball. He shared with us that his previous self would have done that. But the practice of kindness held him back. He looked at the man and walked away, saying, "Apologies for the inconvenience, Sir. I wish you well."

He reached out to my team, thanking us for saving him from a very embarrassing aggravation. I feel it only happened because he had been practicing the skills and was thus laying the brain networks to help contain and redirect his anger.

For many years, I have been practicing looking at others, assuming they all have a pure Esse within them (this was the third practice I shared with Dr. German). A helpful byproduct is that when I do not judge people, I do not feel judged by them. This combination (looking at others' essence and not feeling judged) has made my work interactions (including online) much more enjoyable. Waiting in grocery checkout lines has become a fun experience, as has working with someone annoying or someone annoyed at me. It has also curbed my social anxiety because I know precisely how to look at people to keep my adrenaline in check. Prior to that, public speaking put my cardiovascular and endocrine systems through an exhausting workout. Not so much now.

We teach our children to eat, walk, talk, sit, swim, bike, read, and numerous other skills. Seldom do we teach them how to look at the world, particularly at other people. I believe the simple practice of remembering to send a silent good wish to others, knowing that everyone is special and struggling, can transform relationships on the planet. In the Resilient Option program, I call it the Kind Attention and practice it every day. It pulls positive energy out of thin air because when you send a good wish to others, you simultaneously send a good wish to yourself. At the end of the day, without anything else being different, if you wished twenty people well, you would feel your day went a little better.

How would you want the world to look at your children, with judgmental or kind attention? I'm sure you would choose the latter. So, here is a simple suggestion. Look at the world the way you want the world to look at your kids.

As a person of science and despite the idea of Esse being a little metaphysical, believing that deep within us is a storehouse of timeless values that we can be proud of gives me hope and energy. For the sake of convenience, I have called it my Esse. You may have encountered a similar concept elsewhere — in philosophy, poetry, or through faith. I am just giving it a central place in our journey toward self-love.

The soul mate you have been awaiting all your life is within you. Waiting for someone from outside to heal your broken heart might be a very long and potentially disappointing wait. You may also have given undeserving power to a world that will stay busy with its own healing for a long time. Realize you are your best healer, eternal friend, and better half. Once this thought becomes your experienced reality, you will never feel lonely again, even on the far side of the moon.

We started that healing journey with Coco the bunny in my patient Donna's lap. After a brief intro to our three relationships (self, others, and purpose), we learned how guilt and shame cause self-rejection, and three steps to overcoming these universal feelings (this isn't guilt worthy, I am not the only one, and I can transform my guilt into something useful).

From there, we moved toward learning how our comparison instinct creates self-worth contingencies that we can overcome by converting hurtful comparisons into helpful ones (through working on intensity, intention, and interpretation).

In exploring self-love, our desired destination, we added some variety by learning about five life limiters to ensure we respect, befriend, and nurture our physical body as we care for our minds.

As you move deeper into self-love, having a model of the self that helps you see, understand, and embrace your imperfections while still loving your purity will take you farther.

Earlier, I used to get confused by what it meant to be compassionate or forgiving toward the self. Since I am extending and receiving forgiveness, who is forgiving whom? Now it is a bit clearer. The pure Esse in me is compassionate toward and forgiving the struggling, work-in-progress Psyche. We will leverage this understanding in the coming sections.

Thank you so much for walking along with me so far. I promise to stay with you all the way, personally testing every concept and skill I share in my own life.

Our journey continues with exploring the three flavors of self-love: self-compassion, self-acceptance, and self-forgiveness. Let's start with the first one, self-compassion.

Self-Compassion

23

What Is Self-Compassion?

> The self-compassionate evaluate their performance by their values and effort, not by success or failure.

Rob was pacing up and down in my office as I walked into the consultation room. "It's good to meet you, Rob. How are you doing?" I opened the conversation.

"How am I doing?" Rob shot back. "I fired four hundred employees a few hours ago."

I braced for a difficult hour.

Rob was stuck in self-blame and all kinds of "what ifs." Our hour-long meeting extended into my lunch and beyond. We discussed performance neuroscience, emotional intelligence, cognitive bias, guilt, shame, compassion, relationships, purpose, and more.

At the end of the visit, just as he was about to leave, Rob said, "I feel worse now."

Surprised, I asked him to expand on his words, half hoping it wasn't me. Perhaps the room's air conditioner was too strong. Increasing someone's stress level isn't a very desirable outcome of a stress resilience consult!

"No, that's not the point," he said. "When I took my job, if I knew all that I learned in the last two hours, maybe we could have avoided the layoffs."

Whether it was the fall of the Roman Empire, the end of the Mauryan dynasty, or the 2008 financial crisis, in every instance I have studied, a decline in values preceded the bigger downfall.

I pray we learn from our past, never ditch our values, and never have to endure widespread suffering again to reclaim our best selves.

Of all the different values ranging from integrity and purpose to generosity and humility, the most critical one that empowers our every pursuit and connection is compassion.

Compassion

Compassion is the positive pole of your relationship with others and yourself. Its practical connotation is "to feel and help alleviate someone's suffering."

$$+$$

| Negative Judgment | No Judgment | Compassion |

Two related words are empathy and sympathy. Empathy is feeling the other person's pain by mirroring their experience. Compassion translates that feeling into action. Sympathy shows concern for the pain, while compassion responds with warmth and caring for the pain.

Studies that have compared empathy with compassion generally show that empathy is associated with negative emotions and the activation of our brain's pain areas. In contrast, compassion leads to positive emotions and activates our brain's reward network.[1-2] Researchers and contemplatives both posit that compassion isn't fatiguing. Thus, the term compassion fatigue is really empathy fatigue.[3]

My suggestion to everyone, particularly those working in the caring profession, is to convert their empathy into compassion through action. That action could be something tangible or could simply send a positive thought or prayer to the person struggling. The EVA model of a compassionate response might help.

EVA

A complete compassionate response has five sequential steps:[4]
1. You notice another person's pain (instead of turning away)
2. You feel their pain (instead of staying numb or apathetic)
3. You validate their pain (instead of denying or considering that they "deserve their pain")
4. You have a desire to help relieve their pain (instead of letting them suffer)
5. You do something to help relieve their pain (instead of not doing anything)

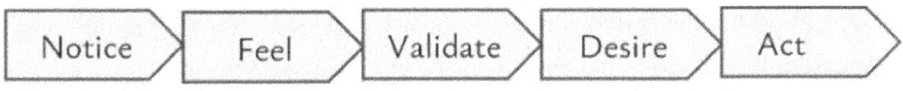

Figure 7: The five steps of self-compassion

1 and 2 together is empathy. 4 and 5 together is action. Thus, my equation for compassion has three components:

Compassion = **E**mpathy + **V**alidation + **A**ction.

The acronym EVA is the Latinate counterpart of Eve, meaning life or full of life. Compassion, indeed, is essential for our species' survival.

Every species has a unique survival strategy. Fish, for instance, lay copious eggs and then leave them to nature. Because of the sheer number, even though a very small percentage (in single digits) survive to adulthood, that's enough to propagate their species. Not so with humans. We produce few, totally dependent offspring. So, we can't move on with life, leaving our newborns to nature. You can blame our phenomenally large brains for that dependence. Here is how that happened.

The brain disadvantage

When our brain was increasing in size, the female pelvis had to expand concurrently to allow safe birth. However, the female pelvis could only expand so much beyond which walking would be difficult. Nature had to make a compromise, which was bringing human newborns into the world with smaller and thus less developed brains. The less developed brains meant very dependent newborns.

Raising a human newborn thus had to be a collective tribal responsibility requiring tremendous cooperation and sacrifice. The force that enables cooperation is compassion. That's why I consider compassion, for others and self, as the mother of all values.

EVA for self

Like compassion for others, self-compassion has three parts:
1. **E**mpathy for self
2. **V**alidating the self
3. **A**ction

Self-compassion comforts you in failures and invites you to be happy and celebratory in success. It is a way of relating with the self, with kindness and patience, both when we are proud of ourselves and also when we are disappointed in the self.

You work very hard to avoid being in the company of mean people. Cultivating self-compassion helps you forever be in the company of a life-affirming presence: your own.

Self-compassion doesn't overlook our imperfections. Instead, it acknowledges our blemishes, knowing many or all of them are a part of being human. Further, self-compassion increases your ability to serve the world; it powers your compassion toward others. Professor Julianne Holt-Lunstad, a career scientist and the lead science editor of the 2023 Surgeon General's Advisory on loneliness, shared with me a few weeks ago, "When we have compassion for ourselves, we are more likely to have compassion for others. This can cyclically reinforce positive social bonds." A large body of research supports her words.

The first step to self-compassion is self-empathy.

Self-empathy

Security guards have one of the highest turnover rates in the industry — between 100 to 300 percent. You can imagine why. Tasked with survival and safety, they must stay constantly alert, draining their nervous system. The same applies to our Psyche.

However, Psyche has it worse. Psyche knows that it will eventually fail in its job, given that we all are mortal. Unlike humans, most animals don't think about their or their loved one's illness, disability, or mortality. We carry health, disability, and life insurance. Some even book an appropriate burial place ahead of time.

Further, your heart beats not just for you. It also beats for the people closest to you. The more you care about people and the more people you care about, the greater your worries. I'm sure you have heard the expression, "You are only as happy as your least happy child."

Even celebratory moments during success tend to be transient; they are quickly followed by a concern that we could lose it all in a blink.

Every human thus needs a healthy helping of self-empathy that involves two processes:

1. You notice your pain
2. You feel your pain

As a self-empathic person, you don't suppress your pain or related thoughts because suppression causes thoughts and feelings to recoil back and stick longer. When you suppress a thought, even though you might seem calm on the outside, the pain and stress areas of your brain (the amygdala and insula) are red hot on the inside.[5] The energy, instead of finding a release, hurts your physical and emotional being. Research shows thought suppression harms your physical health, memory, and relationships, and worsens your mood.[6-8]

Engaging with pain, however, doesn't mean you identify so much with your pain that you become fused with it. You won't enjoy your company if you can't separate your pain from your self. Instead, notice your struggles and watch them like watching your life as a movie.

Watching a movie feels different and less intrusive than being in the movie. Pain becomes less painful just by being noticed and acknowledged. Thus, self-empathy helps you become comfortable experiencing your negative emotions, as long as these emotions do not cause sustained or severe melancholia or anxiety.

Young children are a perfect example of healing through feeling. When they must cry, they hold nothing back. The entire biosphere around them vibrates to the tune of their vocal cords. But the moment you find their purple pony, it's all better. The smile is back, even though the cheeks are still wet with the salty tears. It reminds me of the sun coming out while it is still raining. They recover so fast in part because they allow their emotions to course through them.

Opening yourself up to noticing and feeling the pain, however, isn't for the faint of the heart. We dread pain and will do anything to avoid it.

So, empathy needs courage. I find that courage from thinking that I am bigger than my pain. Through faith, philosophy, neuroscience, or based on what I have shared, if you believe in the presence of an inner pure sacred unblemishable Esse, then you can "look at" your pain and feel it from that place without fear or deep hurt.

Between noticing and feeling the pain and healing it, a big wall of judgment stands, often erected by the world. Of the many patients with chronic pain I have seen, I can group them into two:

1. Those who judged themselves or felt judged by others,
2. Those who did not judge themselves and didn't feel judged by others.

The first group does much better in the long term (lower pain and better well-being) than the second group.

Self-validation

A self-validating person doesn't judge their Psyche's worries, knowing that their Psyche, like every other human, has a complex, almost impossible task of securing the well-being of every life form and the inanimate that the Psyche cares about. For many of us, our definition of self expands to include our home, company, automobile, financial savings, precious belongings, and a societal cause. Children are particularly vulnerable to spells of grumpiness when losing their favorite toy.

As you grow emotionally and in wisdom, fewer objects enter your definition of self. Keep in mind, though, that wisdom and age are not necessarily correlated.[9-10] I'm sure you have encountered some grownups who act like four-year-olds!

A self-validating person also recognizes that the task of theirs and their fellow humans has become increasingly arduous due to the world's growing complexity. To execute its task, your Psyche is neither a perfect tool nor fully equipped. It has biases and blind spots, it sometimes gets greedy or irrationally fearful, and despite meaning well, Psyche finds it challenging to resist short-term gratifications. No wonder the most devout believers philander at times, have a hot mic moment, or get carried away in an argument with the neighbor.

We engage in these behaviors partly because, during our formative years, we saw adults do the same. We created life scripts based on our interpretations of external messages. Those life scripts, right or wrong, now drive our instincts. Every time we think, speak, or act based on those scripts, we make them stronger.

Strong life scripts can be the basis for triggers that generate an outsized response to our circumstances. Triggers can control our minds, at least for the short term. Sometimes, walking upstream on your triggers can tell a lot about your repressed past that needs healing.

As you know, your repressed past was created because, as a child, you critically depended on others for self-evaluation, forcing you to conform to the prevailing norms around you. So, even though you created your life scripts, you didn't *really* cause them. Won't that awareness evoke self-validation and thus, self-compassion?

Compassion to others = Compassion to self

One of the most memorable moments of my life was dialoguing with His Holiness Dalai Lama, listening to his stories and infectious laughter. One of the stories he shared was about a monk who was in prison for over two decades. After finally escaping, the monk went to Dharamshala to meet His Holiness.

Shortly after they hugged, Dalai Lama asked, "Were you afraid in the prison?"

The monk nodded in the affirmative.

"Were you afraid of torture by the prison guards?" Dalai Lama asked.

"No," the monk said.

"Then what were you afraid of?"

"I was afraid I would lose my compassion for the guards."

His commitment to compassion for others did wonders to protect his mental health during one of the most trying times a human can face.

In personal development, we often discuss the difference between state and stage. State is your temporary "state of being," such as sleep. You move from one state to another, sometimes several times a day. Stage is a one-way change that is permanent. It is an irreversible evolution of who you are. For example, once you are an adult, you won't be a toddler again.

When we grow in life, we often change in state, like a ball being rolled up the mountain. It rolls back the moment you stop pushing. Through our growth, a time comes when we won't roll back again. We are transformed. Having gone past the cliff, we have permanently changed. The monk was a breathing embodiment of compassion. No ordinary life situation could move him to compromise his values.

For that transformation, try to commit yourself to your values all day, all week, all month, all year round. A time will come when compassion will be as natural to you as your breath. You'll then be like a sage, healing the world and yourself.

So far, we have discovered the first two self-compassion steps: self-empathy and self-validation. Before we move to the third step, Action, a word of caution is in order.

Recently, I was speaking to employees of one of the biggest financial companies in the world. I sensed a lot of resistance among the approximately 800 participants with embracing positivity. Many assumed self-compassion and self-acceptance will make them lose their edge. I totally see their point but also feel that's a perfect way to push positivity away.

It took me some time to convince them that self-compassion doesn't mean shirking responsibility, excessive self-indulgence, an easy pass, or lowering standards. Confusing self-compassion for weakness or softness is one of the biggest barriers people face in their journey toward being kind to themselves. Let's understand all the different barriers to dismantle them.

24

Common Barriers to Self-Compassion

> The warmth that we feel in a blanket comes from within us.

Several years ago, a colleague asked me to see Jerry, a middle-aged gentleman with early-stage thyroid cancer. Jerry's cancer was curable, but he had declined all treatments. The referring physician warned me to anticipate a difficult visit.

When I met him, Jerry seemed like a perfectly reasonable person. However, the moment we discussed his thyroid cancer, Jerry's face tensed up, wrists clenched, and ears turned red. He seemed ready to jump across the table. Remembering my commitment to "Assuming Positive Intent," I tried my best to stay calm and invited him to share his reservations.

"I lost my sister to a doctor's greed," Jerry said.

I responded with an open invitation. "I am really sorry about what happened to your sister. Do you wish to share more?"

Jerry then elaborated how his sister received an unneeded procedure for a pancreatic cyst, which started a chain of events leading to her untimely passing.

I sensed that Jerry's mind block wasn't a lack of awareness of what to do for his cancer. His main challenge was a lack of trust. He carried a bias that the health systems care mainly about money, with everything else being secondary. So, after saying something like, "I would also be very concerned if I believed that," I shared the compensation system in my hospital, which was based on a fixed salary, and did not offer any performance-based incentives.

"Are you saying my doctor wouldn't get a single extra dollar for taking out my thyroid?" Jerry asked, his eyes wide in disbelief. This was news to him.

"Yes, that's correct," I said.

Once Jerry learned that his surgeon was purely interested in his welfare, he willingly enlisted for the procedure.

Our misguided beliefs

Sometimes, we carry biases that prevent us from seeing the truth. The resulting misguided words and actions could harm us. For instance, research shows the more negative beliefs we carry about self-compassion and ourselves, the less likely we are to be compassionate to the self.[1] Let us look at some common myths about being kind to the self and what research says about them.

Myth #1. I don't deserve self-compassion

"You are a waste of our DNA." Jill, a philanthropist and a brilliant entrepreneur repeatedly heard these words from her parents for standing up to them. When the verbal assaults escalated into physical abuse, she ran away from home. While living in halfway homes, she continued her studies at a state college and married an amazingly loving man with whom she built a phenomenally successful business empire.

Yet, despite living a modest life and contributing millions to charitable causes, Jill feels unworthy and undeserving. "I feel like a selfish freeloader who got way more than she deserved," she said one day. Her success and the love she got from the world as an adult has done little to heal her inner loneliness. Caught in her parents' dark shadows, she doesn't feel she deserves self-compassion.[2]

Myth #2. Self-compassion is just a made-up idea with no real benefits

Over a hundred studies support the benefits of self-compassion. The price of being low on self-compassion isn't just worse mental health, burnout, and fatigue.[3] It is also worse self-care (smoking, unhealthy eating, lack of exercise), less happiness, hope, and life satisfaction, and poorer physical health.[4-5] As one of my colleagues said, "Self-compassion is at the cutting edge of science." I would add to that, "If self-compassion was a pill, I would take it four times a day for the rest of my life!" Dr. Jonathan Fisher, cardiologist and bestselling author of, *Just One Heart*, agrees. In a recent communication, he wrote to me, "Connection begins within, as we extend love from our hearts to the wounded parts of ourselves. Self-compassion not only nurtures our own well-being, but it also has a powerful spillover effect, enriching our relationships with others and creating a ripple of kindness and connection."

Myth #3. I will become a weaker person with self-compassion

The chemicals in poison ivy cause little direct harm right away. The nastiest inflammation happens a few hours later because of the body's immune response to the initial exposure. The same happens with a traumatic experience causing enduring stress.

Self-compassion provides a stop to this simmering stress, which decreases the risk of post-traumatic stress disorder (PTSD), shifting instead to post-traumatic growth.[6] In several medical conditions (such as chronic pain, diabetes, and cancer) and life challenges (such as domestic violence, divorce, natural disasters, and dealing with prejudice), self-compassion empowers the individual for better coping and change.[7]

Dr. Gurmeet Narang, a humanitarian and an awardee from the World Happiness Congress, had all but given up on life after losing his son, wife, and then his daughter over a span of a few years. Devastated and alone, he shared with me how self-compassion helped him find a path to his purpose: "Self-compassion helped me find a way to hold my own struggles and sorrows in my heart while seeing the light of wisdom revealed from my wounds. I realized that as others are important to me, I am also important to me. I found my healing, enabling me to reach out to others who might be alone in their suffering." I have no doubt that self-compassion served as a source of strength to Dr. Narang, transforming him into a global happiness ambassador.

Myth #4. People high on self-compassion act selfish

The assumption that self = selfishness and compassion = weakness couldn't be further from the truth. Imagine you have a pot of compassion energy within you. The fuller the pot, the more you can share with others.

Do you think practicing self-compassion would empty or fill this pot? Research shows it will fill it. When you are content within yourself, you are content with the world.

The more compassion you give to yourself, the more compassion you have within you to give to others. For over two decades, my colleague and resilience researcher, Dr. Sherry Chesak, has been practicing and teaching self-compassion to nurses who feel overwhelmed with compassion fatigue and burnout. She said, "In my years of helping nurses, I find that those who practice self-compassion are best equipped to extend genuine compassion to others." Research fully supports Dr. Chesak's experience. Several studies show that self-compassionate healthcare professionals and first responders find greater satisfaction in helping others and have a lower risk of burnout.[8-9] Self-compassion helps you include yourself without excluding others.

Among couples, the greater their self-compassion, the more emotionally connected and accepting and less aggressive and controlling they are.[10] These traits, along with greater forgiveness and better perspective-taking that occur concurrently with self-compassion, enhance the quality of your relationships.[11] In several other situations where altruism is needed, such as helping others in emergencies and managing interpersonal conflicts, individuals with high self-compassion tend to perform better.[12]

Finally, the self-compassionate people also become more moral. For example, people who learn self-compassion are more likely to accept their mistakes, apologize, and not repeat their transgressing behavior.[13]

Myth #5. Self-compassion might take away my motivation

When self-compassion was first described, researchers equated it with a gentle, tender approach to relating with the self. Building on her earlier work, Dr. Kristin Neff, the pioneering self-compassion researcher, has proposed a new, fiercer kind of self-compassion, one equated with a mama bear when she is protecting her cubs.[14] It combines courage, speaking up, saying No, and even being harsh to unkind people if that's what the situation merits. Thus, self-compassion motivates one to preserve self-love, even if that entails a firm and assertive stance.

Students who once failed an exam performed significantly better the second time around when they worked on self-compassion to combat their previous failure.[15] Another study showed that self-compassion also decreased their fear of failure.[16]

Additionally, concurrent with better performance, students with greater self-compassion cared more about the meaning of their striving compared to just success.[17]

The wiser pursuit in life helps you let go of frivolous goals. Thus, self-compassionate people are less likely to be excessively perfectionistic and focus less on superficial goals (such as fame); instead, they think more about personal mastery.[18]

Myth #6. The more self-compassionate I become, the more I will indulge myself, hurting my health

A particular challenge today is resisting temptations such as calorie-dense food, smoking, stimulating agents, and comforts that predispose to sedentary living. A brain that adapted to food insecurity yesterday must now protect its owner from caloric excess. That's a tall order but essential because many short-term pleasurable activities can hurt us long-term.

Opposite to indulgence, self-compassion protects you from temptations by improving your self-regulation.[19] As a research article mentions, "When people care about themselves, they will care for themselves."[20] Further, self-compassion gives you double the benefit because you are both the receiver and giver of compassion.

The right behaviors often need us to overcome a short-term unpleasant hump. As a self-compassionate person, you are willing to seek the unpleasant, such as the fatigue of exercise or the awkwardness of taking the blame where it is due. You gracefully accept critique, embodying the persona of a humble student. You focus on what it will take to heal and transform you long-term. You think about what's right, not what you want now or what is pleasant, which may or may not be right. That, in essence, is the practice of self-compassion.

Ronaldo sings to his grandma

Ronaldo felt he had failed everyone. He was a famed opera singer with a "one in a billion voice," that could give you goosebumps even on a hot summer day. But for the past six months, his voice had increasingly turned hoarse. A skilled team of doctors sorted out all his medical issues, but he still couldn't find his tenor. Ronaldo's band depended on him, his wife admired his singing, his family needed his financial support, and singing was the gift that had brought him out of drugs. He was spiraling down, living on coke and chips, worried he might go back to the white powder.

He had gained forty pounds in three months. Psychiatrists, however, didn't think he fulfilled the criteria for any mood disorder.

"I am worthless. I am an idiot. I sound worse than a crow," he said to me.

"You have many identities, Ronaldo. You are a husband, a dad, a son, a brother, a grandson, a friend, a colleague, and a singer. Only one of your identities isn't up to par right now, and that too for a short time. Could you be hurting all your other relationships by focusing on just one struggling aspect of your life and that too a transient struggle?"

Ronaldo paused. Something about what I shared made sense to him.

"Maybe you could stop thinking about yourself as a singer for a few months. Nurture other aspects of your life." I shared a few specific resilience practices with him (similar to Dr. German) and asked him to come again in about eight weeks.[21]

About three months later I saw Ronaldo again. "It has been a year since I laughed so hard," Ronaldo said. "But I still can't sing."

"Great to hear the first part. Tell me, what happens when you sing?"

"I start well. But then I feel judged. I feel my audience isn't satisfied with my performance. I start worrying my voice will crack. I overthink. I leave everyone dissatisfied."

"Who loves you unconditionally, Ronaldo? Think about someone who believes in you, in whose presence it won't matter even if your voice cracked."

"My grandma," he said, without thinking for a moment.

"Tell me more."

"Even as an adult, I would put my head in her lap, and she would stroke my hair. All my stress would melt away in her presence."

"How about singing to your grandma? Request her to be in the audience each time you perform. Sing for her."

"But she is no more."

"Then have an extra chair in the audience that you leave empty. Imagine her spirit is present on that chair." Ronaldo's eyes brightened.

A few months later I saw him again, this time for a brief 15-minute follow-up. That was a good sign.

"I'm back," he said with a firm handshake. "Just came to give you my CD and a hug. I sing for my grandma every time, and she is loving it!"

Ronaldo needed to believe in himself, fall in love with his voice again, reclaim a positive, nurturing inner connection, and be in a presence where he was accepted and loved for who he was without any expectations. He needed to be compassionate to himself.

In the next three chapters, we will explore three levels of self-compassion, the reason why we do not trust ourselves, and the very important topic of imposter syndrome (I prefer to call it Imposter Phenomenon. Why give another diagnostic label to a common human experience?).

This discussion will be a prelude to the final two chapters of this longer section — insights and practices (Action) that help with self-compassion.

25
Three Levels

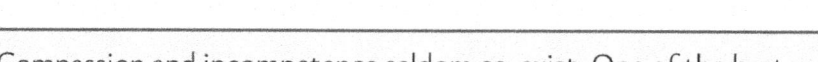

> Compassion and incompetence seldom co-exist. One of the best ways to enhance performance is to build compassion, for others and self.

Just as stepping on a nail predictably hurts your feet, seeing other's pain similarly activates your brain's sensory and emotional areas (the pain matrix). The extent of activation correlates with your level of compassion.[1-2] In other words, your brain looks at someone else's pain as yours.

A fascinating study looked at brain activation in response to observing the pain of others among recent immigrants to Australia. When new immigrants saw people from their race experiencing the pain, their brain areas turned red and purple. However, seeing the locals in pain created minimal activation. With time, this differential decreased as the immigrants assimilated with the locals. Further, their racial bias decreased the most when they got to know others in everyday life.[3]

The above study provides us with three conclusions:
1. We all have a capacity for compassion.
2. We implicitly create exclusions for our compassion.
3. With greater familiarity, these exclusions become less prominent.

Completely excluding a group of people from compassion has led to the inhumane treatment of prisoners of war, undocumented immigrants, and poverty-stricken people, all the way to the genocides that continue to pockmark twenty-first-century history. Similarly, completely excluding the self from compassion leads to low self-worth, shame, depression, disconnection, and eventually thoughts and actions of self-harm.

A vast majority of people who die by suicide (700,00 every year; one person every forty seconds) haven't done anything cruel to feel so low and hopeless. The same applies to millions (likely billions) who contemplate self-harm or experience depression or burnout. That is the reason I suggest removing all exclusions and contingencies as the first step to self-compassion. The three levels I mention next provide a rough track of progression in self-compassion. See where you are presently and what steps you can take to move to the next level.

Three levels of self-compassion

My friend Karina becomes defensive at the slightest perception of her mistake. A simple statement by her son, "The tortilla seems a little burnt," would start her on a self-rejection monologue. "You see, I can't even make a good tortilla anymore. In fact, I was never good at cooking. I also forget everything. Look at the sagging skin under my arms. I think I am falling apart." And on and on. Karina struggles with a lack of self-compassion.

You must be very careful with your words when talking to people who are low on self-compassion, lest you hurt them.

Below is a simple, non-validated self-compassion scale I use that can be helpful. You'll notice that each higher level decreases contingencies for self-compassion. I am describing levels 1, 5, and 10 below. Please give yourself a number where you think you are presently so you can work on moving forward.

Level 1: Hard on self ("I am not kind to me")
Struggle with low self-worth, self-respect, and self-love at baseline; can't make or trust friends; easily pushed into prolonged self-blame and self-rejection; avoids taking challenges for fear of failure.

Level 5: Good to self but have limited reserves ("I am kind to me when I am good")
Generally balanced at baseline but sensitive to rejection, blame, criticism, and perception of physical unattractiveness; good at friendships but carry

lingering doubts about relationships; takes challenges but withdraws quickly if risking failure.

Level 10: Good to self and have moderate to high reserve ("I am always kind to me")

Anchored in intrinsic self-worth; looks at criticism, rejection, and blame as an opportunity to grow; takes good care of self; doesn't feel conscious about physical appearance; has enduring and trusting relationships; takes many challenges and persists despite failures.

Based on the above descriptors, where would you place your present level of self-compassion?

1	5	10
Low self-worth	Contingent self-worth	Unconditional self-worth
Low self-respect	Contingent self-respect	Unconditional self-respect
Low self-love	Contingent self-love	Unconditional self-love
Can't make friends	Insecure with friends	Secure with friends
Prone to enduring self-blame	Recover from self-blame	Recover from self-blame
Avoid taking challenges	Withdraw from challenges	Persist despite failures

I started at levels 1-2 as a child. With a neurologic condition, a weak immune system, in the bottom ten percentile for academic achievement, and finding myself unattractive, I didn't have much going for me. This was despite having wonderfully caring parents and siblings. Their loving attention just ricocheted off my surface.

By medical school, I had gradually worked myself to levels 4-5. This was through lots of self-help and spiritual reading, mentorship from my teachers, academic success, and the loving support of my family.

I am most fortunate that now I toggle between levels 6 and 8 partly because of my patients, students, loved ones, and colleagues. Each of them gives me a purpose to get out of bed in the morning and keep striving.

My progress in self-compassion has been slow. It took me four decades to move past level 5, with lots of unneeded suffering along the path. My hope is for you to progress much faster if you are presently scoring lower. I have seen that many times, through a combination of insights and practices that are all embellished with self-trust.

I recently asked my previous colleague, Dr. Jennifer Posa, current chief well-being officer for the Central Intelligence Agency (CIA), for her thoughts on the value of self-compassion at work. In her words, "Self-compassion is a skill that enables one's resilience and readiness. For leaders, and high performing teams, it is especially impactful and best shown when giving grace to others in times of challenge, opportunity, change, and transition."

It is heartwarming to learn that leaders at some of the most cutting-edge organizations recognize the value of self-compassion and integrate it into their approach to well-being.

26

Self-Trust

> If nature can convert dirt into fruits, we can convert hurts into blessings.

"**K**idney disease, heart failure, hepatitis, I must have something," Ralph pleaded.

"Fortunately, all your blood tests and the MRI scan came back negative," I reassured Ralph, to which he responded with a loud, dejected exhalation. "So, you are telling me I am making it all up. It's all in my head."

Ralph was a fifty-eight-year-old father of three who had chronic, unremitting fatigue with bouts of whole-body aches. As a client relations manager, he was a gregarious, high-performing executive known for his upbeat attitude at work. But by the time he got home, he felt like he had been beaten up by a baseball bat after running a double marathon. His fatigue and pain were slowly swallowing his life and what was left of his pride. He could no longer garden, play badminton with buddies, or coach high school soccer. But the worst were the helpless shrugs and sighs of his wife, Mindy, who had to manage the entire house alone. She missed him while he was still around.

Ralph could not trust his body anymore. Nor could he trust his mind. A few years ago, two or three drinks wouldn't bother him. But now, just one drink launched him into an embarrassing monologue often punctuated with curse words.

Ralph was caught in a downward spiral of losing self-trust, a core ingredient that helps us feel confident and effective and is essential for self-compassion.

Self-trust

Am I good enough? Do I sound confident but not overly confident? Do I have what it takes to fulfill this role? Will I be able to manage the crisis that will eventually come? Am I as good as people think? No one knows the perfect answer to these questions, but your positive beliefs about yourself give you hope and enhance your performance. Self-trust is having confidence in your abilities and values.[1]

Self-trust isn't a state of delusion. It doesn't mean believing that you'll always win. Instead, self-trust is a conviction that you will give it your best. Similarly, self-trust doesn't mean you'll always stay positive and do the right thing. It means you won't turn away from the negative, will be kind to yourself through success and failure, and instead of avoiding looking at your mistakes, you will meet them with the perspective of a student, so you do not repeat them.

In self-trust, like other engagements with the self, you are both extending and receiving the trust.

We don't trust ourselves when we only focus on our lower tendencies. Self-trust emerges from awareness of Esse and Psyche, recognizing that just as we are a work in progress, deep within us is an ambrosia of wisdom waiting to be accessed.

As you might imagine, this awareness isn't intuitive for many of us. The world also does a great job of dismantling our self-trust very soon after we arrive.

Instinctive self-doubt

Our default is to doubt our abilities, and for a good reason. Suppose you are a bricklayer, housekeeper, or coin laundry operator whose task is simple, repetitive, and easily protocolized. In that case, how likely are you to feel shaky about your capabilities?

On the other hand, suppose you write lyrics, present keynotes, publish scientific papers, perform surgeries, create music, or engage in any task where you must depend on your non-dependable brain's creativity and endurance. Research shows you're much more likely to have self-doubt in some of these professions.[2-3]

Our brain simply cannot guarantee a consistent output because of the numerous factors that influence its performance. A positive performance keeps us steady, while a negative performance takes us ten notches down, particularly so for our children.

Our disadvantaged children

Many factors come together to put our children at a distinct disadvantage when it comes to building self-trust. Parenting has evolved to increasingly enable children instead of challenging them. Every time we enable a child we decrease their self-trust. We also decimate their self-trust when we are overly critical.[4] Well-meaning parents sometimes say words that decrease kids' trust in their emotions, insights, and decisions. "That is the stupidest thing I have heard." "Only a fool will do what you just did." "Strong kids don't cry."

Neurologically, young children's fear network matures much before their higher cortical brain, which is nature's way of protecting them and providing a greater final level of emotional maturity among adult humans.[5] However, unmitigated fear at a young age interferes with developing self-trust.

Comparisons, particularly upward social comparisons, don't help either. Anyone who spends a few hours on social media daily is unlikely to walk away feeling worthy and self-trusting. Living on comparisons, which now populate every hour of children's awake moments, and self-trust just don't go together.

Of all the different animal species, only humans have parenting practices that dismantle self-trust. Think what would happen if a lion cub never joined a hunt because of their parental fear. Will they ever be able to enter or lead a pride? Or, every time the hunt fails, the dominant male lion takes it out on the younger members. That wouldn't bode well for raising confident, self-trusting, capable cubs. I worry many of our children face one or the other extreme, which hurts their self-trust, a vulnerability we must reverse.

Our early life experiences often force us to grow up with intense pressure to conform and to find satisfaction through pleasing others. Such pressure as an adult might work fine in a mutually loving and caring relationship. But if you live with a selfish, predatory person, they will demand their priorities are met every single day. It is in their interest that you conform by doubting your abilities. Once you yield, entrapping yourself in self-doubt, finding freedom will take a considerable effort.

At work, a lack of self-trust can lead to the widely understood phenomenon of imposter syndrome (or imposter phenomenon).

27
Imposter Phenomenon

> Others see you as they are not as you are. So, the likelihood that everyone will adore you is zero.

Some of us are too intelligent and driven to be happy. The more we challenge our brain, the higher our likelihood of doubting our brain's abilities.

In an interesting paradox, the better your brain's cognitive capacity (thinking, reasoning, memory, language), the greater its emotional vulnerability. You become very good at poking holes in your success. That's why many high-achieving individuals (up to 80 percent) distrust their intellect, skills, or accomplishments.[1] Their contributions flow off their head like the rainwater flows off the concrete. They live in perpetual fear of being exposed as frauds, often experiencing depression and anxiety. These are the self-appointed imposters, walking around universities, hospitals, and other campuses, giving their best and more, yet feeling miserable.

Many have a need (not just a desire) to be the best, turning them into hyper-competitive perfectionists. They have two specific phobias: atychiphobia (fear of failure) and achievemephobia (fear of success).

The fear of failure makes sense, but why would anyone fear success? It's because they worry that their success will create higher future expectations that they cannot meet. How sad that some of our society's most brilliant and hardworking members experience the most suffering at their own hands.[2-4]

I so wish we get more SUAVE about trusting ourselves so we can evict the imposter within us. The word suave means polished, smooth, and able to deftly handle relationship nuances, including with the self. For now, consider it an acronym for a five-component approach to enhance self-trust and manage moments you feel like an imposter. The five components are Self-aware, Upskilled, Adventurous, Values-centric, and Equipoised.

Self-aware

In our present state of evolution, we have limited awareness of our physical body, emotional state, or where we are going.

For instance, as a physician, I have seen many patients who had moderate anemia, kidney or liver failure, or a weak heart muscle, but they had zero or minimal symptoms. The brain sensors that monitor our internal physical state aren't sensitive enough or easily trainable.[5]

The same applies to our minds. "I had no idea I was so stressed" is a common expression I hear from people once they get past a challenging phase of their life. A little over 10 percent carry a diagnosis called Alexithymia. People with Alexithymia are considered "emotionally blind" since they can't feel their emotions very well.[6]

Two-thirds of us lack clarity about our life's purpose or direction.[7-8] Many of us aren't aware of the repressed memories and rejected part of us that we carry in our Psyche.

Becoming more self-aware starts you on a path to know yourself better, an early step in building your self-trust. A thoughtful response to some of the following questions might enhance your self-awareness:

- What are my strengths and weaknesses?
- What do I really care about?
- What do I like, and what do I detest?
- When do I feel content?
- What am I proud of?
- What embarrasses me the most?
- What do I need to be at my best?
- What obstacles have I overcome in the past?
- Do I have any specific regrets?
- What are my top worries?

A simple grounding practice I sometimes do these days is to pause in the middle of the day for two minutes and recap all that has transpired since I woke up. I also think about my purpose and the good people in my life. I might do a similar practice at night. In this practice, I find areas of learning and growth, moments that nurture me, and some that might need healing. Thinking about all I have tackled today gives me trust that I can do the same and some more tomorrow. It also gives me a feeling of accomplishment and control.

Reeva Misra, founder and CEO of WONE, a highly successful AI powered workplace well-being platform, knows fully well the importance of a healthy connection with self, others, and purpose for an entrepreneur who must negotiate new terrains every day. She told me, "An entrepreneur's journey can be cited as lonely and uncertain as you're creating a future that hasn't been seen before. Connecting deep within to a purpose much larger than myself has allowed me to deepen my relationship with myself, with others on a similar path and bond more strongly with a shared mission."

An important reminder here is that we learn most life lessons after repeating the same mistake several times, not just once. So, do not blame yourself for stubbing your toe on the same ledge over and over.

Finally, an essential part of self-awareness is reminding ourselves that our self is a combination of the vulnerable, ever-changing Psyche and the ever-pure, unchanging Esse. While not essential to self-awareness, believing in one's innate purity could be a vital resource for coping with life's most challenging moments. Let your mind see the light that your eyes can't see.

Upskilled

Let's consider two situations where your car is at 50 mph. In one instance, you are accelerating toward 70 mph, while in another instance, you are decelerating toward 25 mph. Which one will feel faster? Most people say the accelerating one, because momentum matters.

A focus on ongoing learning gives you a sense of accomplishment, growth, and confidence. Learning new things is essential to effectively use what you already know.

Curiosity powers your leaning. The more curiosity you cultivate, the greater your self-trust and lower your imposter feelings. Curiosity does wonders for your brain and may even protect you from dementia.[9-10]

Consider learning at least one new weekly insight that ups your physical, cognitive, emotional, social, and spiritual knowledge. Do consider exploring the following questions:

- How do I increase my health span and play span?
- What is the role of micronutrients for healthy immunity?
- What is working memory, and how can I expand it?
- Why might chasing happiness make one less happy?
- What is the effect of loneliness on my genetic expression?
- What is the relationship between spirituality and brain health?

As you upskill yourself, you will become curious about other aspects of your life.

- Am I doing things that are not a good use of my time?
- What kind of people energize me, and who pulls me down?
- What is my inner critic telling me? Can I hear its voice even if I do not have to buy into it?

Greater self-awareness might help you realize that many people are simultaneously amazing and annoying (I didn't say amazingly annoying!). How you feel about them depends on the aspect you are focusing on.

Once, Richa and I were frustrated with a loved one. After a few minutes of venting, when guilt took over, we made a list of all that was good about that person. Since that day, I have seen that person in a very different light.

Adventurous

Your foray into better self-awareness and upskilling increases your self-trust, resulting in an uptick in your ability to handle uncertainty. You become more open to change. You start taking novel detours instead of following an already-paved path.[11]

Courage is often misunderstood. Standing on the battlefield fighting the bad guys indeed takes courage. Creating an entirely new dish in the kitchen for a picky family also takes courage. So does going out and talking to people despite social anxiety, donating blood despite having needle phobia, standing in front of a class to talk about your research project, and taking the driving test even though you failed the first two times.

Courage isn't the absence of fear; it is the presence of love. Courage prompts you to do the right thing despite the fear. The courageous pursue purpose instead of evading failure. The anxious and the underprivileged are often more courageous than those endowed with a calm mind, riches, and choices.

With every micro risk you take, your self-trust improves, particularly when you do not give up. If you succeed, your self-trust doubles. If you fail, you carefully examine the cause of failure. Your ability to examine failure instead of putting yourself down by itself improves your imposter feelings.

One area where I miserably failed after I arrived in the U.S. was driving. My first pre-GPS, $500 car wasn't the easiest to steer. Thankfully, I never crashed, but I frequently lost my way. With a stiff steering wheel and a medieval side mirror, I wasn't very comfortable changing lanes on the highway, so I would drive in the right lane. Eventually, it would become the exit lane, forcing me to take an unplanned exit. Invariably, I would arrive in an unknown neighborhood and make a U-turn from the cul-de-sac. I began keeping 30 minutes of "getting lost time" for every trip!

Richa and I then made some changes. We mapped drives ahead of time, planned every drive together, and identified landmarks at which to change lanes. My comfort and skill improved. I also eventually bought a new car with the GPS installed.

The GPS was a game changer. I could now trust myself to find my way no matter how lost. I became more adventurous, choosing to lose my way a few times just for fun, and even drove two thousand miles across the U.S.

While developing the Resilient Option program, I created a values-based GPS for my mind that has helped me better negotiate the tortuous and confusing world of emotions. I feel privileged to share that with you next.

Values-centric (My mind's GPS)

About two decades ago, while working on an approach to build resilience, I learned about the power and weaknesses of the human brain. I envisioned two brain loops — the limbic loop and the cortical loop that I shared with you earlier. The limbic loop is the reactive, fear and greed-driven system riddled with biases, constant doubts, and worries. Many longstanding traumas are stored in the limbic loop. From this storage, the traumas intermittently resurface as strong sensitivities.

The cortical loop is more responsive and values-driven, seeks the truth, and is thus comfortable with uncertainty. I recognized that I spent much of my days in the instinctive limbic loop. With better awareness, I tried to switch my loop by creating a GPS for my mind with values that engage the prefrontal cortex.

My mind's GPS (GPS-m) has five values: gratitude, compassion, acceptance, meaning, and forgiveness. Each weekday has its value in the following schematic, with Saturday and Sunday focused on celebration and reflection/prayer. (Table 2)

Table 2. A set of values to redirect the mind

Monday	Gratitude
Tuesday	Compassion
Wednesday	Acceptance
Thursday	Meaning
Friday	Forgiveness
Saturday	Celebration
Sunday	Reflection / Prayer

Here are two ways to use GPS-m:

1. As a <u>responsive measure</u>, when already amidst a difficulty, use the day's go-to thought to realign your perspective. For example,

On Monday: What went right in what went wrong? (to recover faster from a loss)
On Tuesday: An expression other than love is a call for help. (to reframe others' annoying behaviors)
On Wednesday: If it won't matter in five years, don't let it matter today.
On Thursday: Could this short-term adversity help your long-term purpose? Which of your actions better aligns with your North Star?

On Friday: Don't let someone who shouldn't be in the story of your life write the title of your story.

2. As a <u>proactive measure</u> to live with greater positivity, keep the assigned value as the guiding principle for the day. Thus, proactively seek greater gratitude on Monday, compassion on Tuesday, etc. Consider reading, writing, thinking, sharing, and practicing that value for the day.

Three ground rules to use GPS-m are:
1. Be flexible. Please don't say, "I can't be compassionate today because it's not a Tuesday!"
2. Try another principle if the first go-to principle for the day doesn't work.
3. Whenever in doubt, try gratitude; if it fails, compassion (including self-compassion).

After a few months of using GPS-m, I began developing greater self-trust (and lower imposter feelings). The result was a greater sense of belonging (at home and work) and saying yes to more opportunities. When stressed or confused, I knew my GPS would put me back on the highway.

Here are a few additional advantages of letting your values dominate your thinking (from my personal experience and that of thousands of my students/clients):

- You have less need for others' approval. Since you trust that the values will steer you in the right direction, you are more confident in your thoughts, words, and actions.[12]

- You are not as affected by competition. Your mindset shifts from scarcity to abundance since you come to believe in the principle of "May the best team win." You are happy with others' successes, even if you didn't succeed.

- You recognize that our Psyche focuses on the pleasant while life's greatest pursuits entail seeking the right. In other words, you eat more lettuce than donuts!

- You make fewer promises but follow through on the ones you make. Your willpower improves, so you are more thoughtful about your pursuits, not letting minor setbacks deter you from your path.

Values have a depth beyond the visibly simple. Gratitude can be for the visible positives in life, but at a deeper level, you can be grateful for each breath, your adversities, and even tomorrow, despite not knowing what it will bring. Such an anchor gives you an inner equipoise from which the strongest tempest and temptations can't budge you.

Equipoised

I worked with a senior researcher on an important initiative a few years ago. He was as amazingly brilliant as he was committed. Before one of our afternoon meetings, he received an ominous diagnosis that was sure to limit his life to a few months. Instead of canceling the two-hour meeting, he remained focused on the task at hand.

Later, he rallied the group to complete the multi-year project in three months. He passed away shortly after the project's completion. I learned so much from him — his love for science, passion for making a difference, and equipoise.

Equipoise is your ability to stay steady and balanced despite perturbations that could derail you. It is not dry neutrality or an "I couldn't care less" attitude. Instead, equipoise is your ability to focus on what matters and is actionable. The confidence that comes from your self-awareness, upskilling, willingness to take risks, and anchor in values gives you the equipoise.

Flexibility and equipoise go together. You are flexible about preferences and firm in principles. You are comfortable being interdependent and bringing out the best in everyone. Such equipoise makes you confident yet humble. Your driving values make you generous, which, combined with confidence and humility, removes hesitation from seeking the right help. Further, you no longer worry about experiencing negative emotions, which helps you take measured risks with less fear.

Such people do not create products, so that they can buy a private island in the Pacific. Their efforts are to serve the world. Their Psyche is now fully serving their Esse. They have integrated and transcended their hurts.

I pray you cultivate greater self-trust every day to develop enduring self-love.

Payal Sahni Becher, Chief People Experience Officer at Pfizer, shared with me a gist of her life's wisdom collected over decades of working with tens of thousands of employees. She said, "I find that a healthy relationship with oneself is essential to overcoming imposter phenomenon. Adversities are inevitable, but when you have resilience and self-love, you find the strength to surf through life's challenges with grace and strength." I completely agree and believe that helping our brains lift a heavier load will be as important as trying to decrease our load in the coming years.

I'll share more insights on the Imposter Phenomenon in the section on Self-Acceptance. Presently, I feel we are ready to move to the fifth step of self-compassion: Action.

Let's work toward cultivating the strength to surf, not sink, by integrating some of the self-compassion insights and practices.

28
Actionable Insights

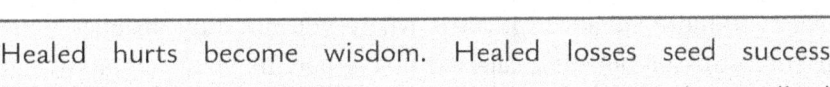

> Healed hurts become wisdom. Healed losses seed success. Remember if you are hurting or losing today that someday you'll call them with different names.

As I start writing this chapter, I feel like we have already covered many of the self-compassion insights. So, instead of discussing the entire breadth, let's focus on five core ideas that are immediately actionable. They are: pinpoint to free, remove contingencies, optimize expectations, tame your amygdala, and let Esse take over.

Pinpoint to free

When a patient comes to me with a fever, I try to pinpoint the problem. Do they have a sore throat? A cough? How is their tummy? Any skin rashes? The goal is to diagnose the precise problem and what body part it is affecting. Even though the patient as a whole has a fever, in someone with pneumonia, the problem is with the lungs.

As we understand ourselves better, we get skilled at isolating the problem. Here are the levels of our progression in this pursuit and how it relates to our relationship with stress and self-compassion:

Level 1: I am stressed

At this level, we can't tell ourselves apart from our stressor. We are vulnerable to generalizing our feelings and shaming ourselves. We feel we "deserve" our negative emotions, fully believing the hurtful rejections stored in our Psyche.

Level 5: I am feeling stressed

Now we have separated ourselves from our stress. We can "see" our Psyche instead of being fused with it. This distancing helps us observe our symptoms with less judgment. Simply dispassionately observing a symptom without any other action gives you the power to better manage the symptom.

Level 10 – My Psyche feels stressed

An even more advanced level is where you not only distance yourself from your stressor but also can see that a part of you, perhaps the most precious part, was, is, and always will remain unblemished. That part of you, your Esse, feels and expresses compassion for your Psyche. Self-compassion no longer feels forced or undeserved.

Based on the above descriptors, where would you place your present relationship with your stressors?

1	5	10

As you advance past level 5, instead of looking at the world with the eyes of stress, you begin to perceive that stress is just a transient disturbance in your Psyche. Stand back and observe, validate, and show your compassion for the part of you that is still vulnerable.

Remove contingencies

When we lived in small tribes, our comparisons were limited to the 150 members of our tribe (called the Dunbar number). Likely, none of the members had the beauty, the brawn, or the brains that might make us feel several logs inferior. That's not so now. With a few clicks, we have the world's best accessible to us to make us feel miserable. Now, with AI-enabled enhancements, all bets are off. Comparisons create contingencies that give our Psyche the fodder it needs to keep us in its hold.

My suggestion is to move forward with optimizing both comparisons and contingencies so you can continue progressing while staying kind to yourself. Below are some milestones you might encounter.

Level 1: Heavy on comparisons and contingencies

In the default instinctive way of living, we confuse greed and dissatisfaction for motivation. We believe that inspiring ourselves through upward comparisons and innovating new self-worth contingencies once the previous ones are no longer relevant is a great way to get more out of life.

Our smiles are forced, celebrations halfhearted, and no matter our success, envy rules our minds. We try to dominate those who give no pushback. Our Psyche is a storehouse of memories that chronicles the rejections we faced when we tried to assert or protect ourselves. Thus, we find ourselves an easy target for our blame, with no place for self-compassion in our being.

Level 5: Moderate and mostly helpful comparisons and contingencies

You are now aware of the rigged game. The more you succeed, the more opportunities and domains for comparisons. Self-worth contingencies are also greater. In this state, success through hard work only worsens the imposter phenomenon.

With better awareness and working on yourself, you transcend these limitations so now your upward comparisons are to feel inspired, and downward comparisons are to evoke compassion and contentment. Your contingencies are fewer and mainly related to your values. You recognize that others will judge you and are okay with that. You do not generalize their feedback to all aspects of you. Instead, you use it to grow. However, despite all the growth, you still struggle with self-compassion at times because the world keeps reminding you of your "imperfections," and you frequently buckled under those reminders in the past.

Level 10: You are free

You are an epitome of confidence and humility. Despite recognizing that you are a work in progress like everyone else, you are internally at peace with yourself. You seldom experience envy and treat everyone equally, including yourself. You are amused by your Psyche's insecurities, recognizing their origins in the shadows of the past. Instead of getting carried away or feeling guilty, you smile at the occasional greed or irrational fear-laden thoughts, seeing those as evidence of being human.

Based on the above descriptors, where are you in your relationship with comparisons and contingencies?

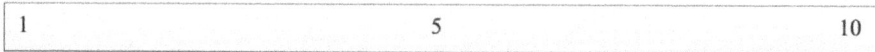

As you advance toward freedom, your key concern is, what is the right thing to do? What would my Esse want? You fully understand that self-compassion helps you focus on the right, not the pleasant. It is a way to do good, not get spoilt. You thus put no limits to self-compassion. You are in love with yourself.

Optimize expectations (of others)

Remember the happiness formula I shared earlier: Happiness = Reality / Expectations. When we are caught in the swirl of comparisons and contingencies, we depend on others to keep filling our leaky bucket. They only have so much to give, and after a point, disengage, which dismantles our sense of self even further.

Eventually, we realize that one of the best ways to keep others close to us is to free them from our expectations or even a commitment to us. This journey, like others, progresses slowly and might be best captured in three descriptors.

Level 1: Unrealistic expectations

Recognize that most of the world is struggling with its demons of low self-worth, loneliness, and excessive stress, which create a preoccupied mind. Depending on a tired person to infuse you with positive energy would be unrealistic.

Earlier in my career, I expected a lot of positive feedback after each presentation. I would take it personally if the participants seemed even the least disengaged. As a result, I kept re-injuring myself, sometimes several times a week. Level 1 isn't a happy place to reside.

Level 5: Realistic expectations

Socks on the floor, clumsily loaded dishwasher, forgotten anniversary, unpaid bills — you smile at your partner's lack of attention to detail instead of getting annoyed. You give them grace through their stressful phase at work. You still have expectations, but increasingly, your hopes are about values rather than mundane inconveniences. In freeing others, you free yourself.

Level 10: Zero expectations

This is unreal and difficult to attain unless you live committed to a life of prayer and service. You not only forgive the past but also forgive the future. I call this preemptive forgiveness. You are like a tree that gives back fruits when people throw rocks at it. You see every person in their fuller context, always assuming positive intent. Your Esse now sees the Esse in every being.

Based on the above descriptors, where are you with respect to your expectations?

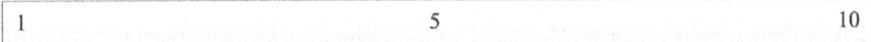

Tame your amygdala

Nature has shortchanged humans in the design of our emotional machinery. Alligators have it easy — no guilt at snapping and drowning an innocent fawn that happens to wander into their territory. Even Zebras have it easier. Within a few minutes of beating a lion in a hundred-meter dash, they are back to nibbling grass. Imagine a human winning that dash? They would have panic attacks, develop generalized anxiety, and need therapy for months.

The reason for this response? Our phenomenal memory system and great imagination. Imagining and experiencing activate the same brain areas.[1] Every time we experience fear, we strengthen those circuits, keeping us locked in the fear loop (one among several positive feedback loops we have discussed in this book). Further, our subconscious storehouse of rejections and repressions can unleash at our most vulnerable moments, often unpredictably.

The beauty is that you have the power to rewire those networks, albeit slowly. Here are the different levels of progression.

Level 1: Amygdala dominant

This is our automatic state where we have a strong fear network that takes over the brain at the slightest perception of threat, physical or emotional, real or imaginary. The release of adrenaline from the initial amygdala activation inhibits the brain's memory and rational areas, particularly the pre-frontal cortex. That's why you can't recall important information when stressed and aren't amenable to rational negotiation when your heart is racing past 120 beats per minute. The result is runaway anxiety that could culminate in a panic attack. In this state, we say no to challenges, connections, and opportunities to protect our emotions.

Level 5: Reactive amygdala that listens to the pre-frontal cortex

Of all the different human predispositions — fear, greed, ego, envy, disgust, anger — fear is often the last one to go. It is because, historically, fear of physical injury has kept us safe.

So, as you grow emotionally and in self-compassion, your amygdala still stays reactive, but increasingly under the influence of your pre-frontal cortex. With fewer and less intense anxious moments, you are more willing to seek novel experiences and risks and connect with new people, thus progressing in life.

Level 10: Dominant pre-frontal cortex with tamed amygdala

You finally arrive at a place where seeing someone angry evokes compassion, not counter anger. Your fears still protect you but do not hold you back. You feel grateful for a glass of water, compassionate toward your demanding supervisor, and can find purpose in the littlest of daily experiences. You balance the long term with the short term, can think through complexity, and embody a healing presence all day. You seldom judge yourself or feel lonely since you are now much more intentional and thrive in your own company.

Based on the above descriptors, where are you in your amygdala-prefrontal cortex balance?

| 1 | 5 | 10 |

Moving from the lower (limbic) to the higher (cortical) areas of the brain occurs concurrently with your Esse taking over your Psyche.

Let Esse take over

As an adolescent, I fancied doing something so substantial that global headline news would cover my work. Looking at the headline news today, I don't fancy that anymore. You can see the play of the very vocal and insecure Psyche on what's happening across the world. Individually, irrespective of the specific path we take, we go through a particular track of progress in our personal evolution.

Level 1: Noisy Psyche silent Esse

Think about someone you know who is selfish, greedy, fearful, immoral, untruthful, and prone to explosive anger. Is this person more likely to dominate the news, or someone selfless, content, moral, truthful, kind, and forgiving? Likely the first one, isn't it? Kindness and forgiveness aren't as newsworthy for the drama-seeking mind. The more extreme the drama, the better. That's why many of us are busy outdoing the other person in how irrational or theatrical we can be to garner attention.

People's attention directly translates to dollars and success in the present world. With Psyche in total control, Esse's gentle whispers, quieter than the heartbeat, fall into the background.

Level 5: Psyche and Esse take turns

You depend significantly on who is with you, like a mirror that reflects its environment. In the presence of kind, values-driven people, you think and speak the truth. But in the presence of entitled ones, you believe you deserve every pleasure coming your way instead of feeling grateful and content. You start building your brain based on your values. You see your brain as a buffet; how you feel depends on the servings you partake of at any moment.

Level 10: Esse takes over

You recognize that you are more than a collection of atoms. You are aware that life is brief and precious. It is a journey to advocate for the lost and the least. You do not worry about being counter-cultural if the prevailing culture doesn't uphold the best values. You disregard the statistic, instead focusing on the person. You do the right thing, always.

Instead of doing big things with little love, you would rather do little things with big love. You respect and dignify human life. Your respect and love are unconditional. You deliberately lower yourself to honor others. This doesn't mean you have low self-worth. Quite the contrary, you are aware of the infinitely precious Esse within you, just as in everybody else.

Based on the above descriptors, how strong is the influence of your Esse on your everyday life?

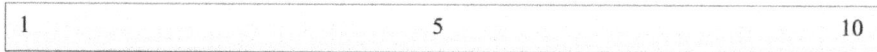

Please look at how you scored in the above five ideas and consider taking concrete steps to advance in areas where you are most struggling. I'll present specific self-compassion skills in the next chapter and build other future materials to help our journey.

Determined Zoe

"This is my final hope," said Zoe, a thirty-year-old sales professional, as she sat in my office. "I have tried every therapy and medicine you can think of. But I still feel like crap. If you can't help me, I will do the ultimate." Zoe's face showed her desperation as well as determination. Not the good kind of determination.

I advised her to continue her therapy and medicines, and after making sure of her safety, provided her insights and practices to transcend her Psyche, which was creating a constant noise in her being.

While I am sure that the therapies Zoe continued significantly contributed to helping her shed her negative symptoms, she ascribes her continued remission to recognizing her Psyche and then developing an acceptance of its vulnerabilities and opening her heart for self-compassion.

Gradually, as she went past the noise, she discovered the silence and then the melody. She felt the desire to share that melody with others, which she is doing now through her business and personal life.

Friend, no one wakes up in the morning thinking, "I am going out to get sad today." No one takes a course in "How to get panic attacks." Most of the emotional hurt and loneliness in the world is unintentional.

Further, we have enough knowledge and resources to take care of everyone. It is a matter of committing to co-creating a world where no one is left alone in suffering. Freeing yourself from negativity, removing contingencies, minimizing expectations, taming your amygdala, and letting your pure essence take over the limited mind can take you to the deepest depths of self-compassion. Pick one of these and take a small step to move closer to 10 (or at least past 5).

Let's hold each other's hands as we walk together, for I need to go there too. Your company will help us both reach further.

As we travel together, let's sing some songs of self-affirmation, take a few deep breaths, and speak words that are uplifting to ourselves and others — all self-compassion practices toward which we turn next.

29
Self-Compassion Practices

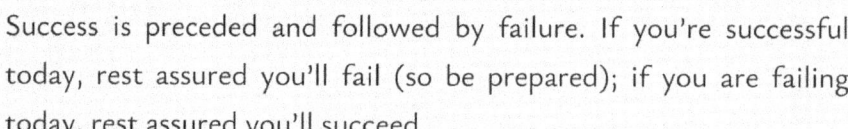

> Success is preceded and followed by failure. If you're successful today, rest assured you'll fail (so be prepared); if you are failing today, rest assured you'll succeed.

Lubdup…….Lubdup……Lubdup…..Lubdup….Lubdup…Lubdup..Lubdup.
Lubdup.Lubdup.Lubdup.Lubdup.Lubdup.Lubdup.Lubdup.Lubdup.Lubdup

I felt my heart thumping as I waited to go live on the NPR. I hadn't slept well the previous night, working with Gauri until 2 a.m. to make a balloon car (the car went forward as the balloon deflated). Now, I feared I would mess up the NPR interview, discrediting me and all those who believed in me. I had a minute or two to gather myself. I closed my eyes and started focusing on exhaling slowly. Then I zoomed out.

I took my awareness above the building I was in to visualize the entire campus, the city, my state, the U.S., planet Earth, the solar system, and finally, the spinning pinwheel of the Milky Way. The awareness of my unimaginably inconsequential presence tucked some 25,000 light years from the galaxy's center gave me peace. My amygdala calmed down; the adrenals slowed their cortisol and adrenaline gush. Everything went well with the interview. Reframing and deep breathing work.

Deep breathing

Our body has neatly parsed the autonomic functions that occur beneath conscious awareness from somatic ones controlled by our will. Thus, you can't do much about the contractions of your gall bladder. This is for a good reason. Imagine having to run your digestive system like you drive your car. You would need to take a two-hour post lunch time out to digest your food! Humans would be so busy running our essential body functions that we would still rub stones to make fire.

However, autonomic and somatic systems overlap at a few places in our body. Breathing is one of them. It is an automatic activity that is also under voluntary control. Breath also provides an opportunity for bidirectional feedback. Here is how it works: When you feel relaxed, your breathing slows; when you intentionally slow your breath, you feel relaxed. Breath thus offers an excellent tool to lower your adrenaline.

Lowering your adrenaline is essential because, as I shared earlier, most rational cognitive strategies stop working during stressful situations when your brain is gorged with excessive adrenaline. That's how stress impairs pre-frontal cortex signaling pathways.[1-3]

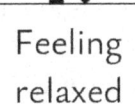

A simple way to practice deep breathing is to make a mental star while taking five deep breaths, with each limb of the star representing one breath. You can take approximately 10 to 12 seconds with each limb, breathing at 5 to 6 breaths per minute.

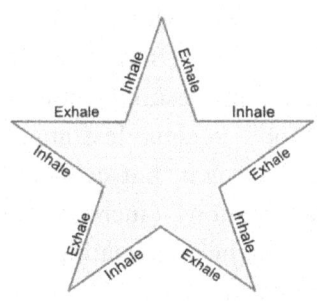

I'm sure you can find countless deep breathing videos on YouTube or other media platforms. The basic idea is to slow your respiratory rate, be intentional about your breaths, and practice longer than normal exhalation to improve the parasympathetic (vagal) activity.[4]

Self-affirmation

Self-affirmation is maintaining a view that you are a good and moral person.[5] Unfortunately, a moment of angry outburst, envious rumination, or any life experience that suggests you are failing in your roles or not living by your values can hurt this positive self-view.

Luckily, many domains collate to create the self-view, including your role as parent, spouse, sibling, friend, colleague, neighbor, and more. You can't get an A+ all the time in each domain. One suggested solution is to "compensate" a failing grade in one domain by crediting your performance in another to maintain a positive self-view. Another approach is through intentional self-affirmation.

For the longest time, I didn't believe in the benefits of positive self-talk, particularly if it was externally mandated and didn't originate in deep inner conviction. Then, I participated in laughter yoga.

Surrounded by several dozen people loudly exhaling "ha ha ha" for no reason, I first found it weird. But gradually, watching other people's laughter, even though I knew it was fake, had an impact. I began laughing and it felt good. Cathartic. Studies proving laughter yoga's effectiveness also helped.[6-8] "If I repeat a thought or experience enough number of times, it starts feeling real," I surmised.

An intriguing series of studies added to my conviction. They originate in what researchers call the facial feedback hypothesis. The hypothesis states that when we see a face, our facial muscles mirror other person's emotion, which helps us understand their internal state.[9] In other words, if we sustain a particular facial expression long enough, we start feeling that way internally.

Researchers next wondered if relaxing the furrowing muscles (corrugator supercilii and the procerus) with agents like botulinum toxin (Botox) would empower us to reduce our anger, fear, and sadness.[10] Interestingly, this is precisely what the studies showed. Not only did people become less angry and happier when Botox took away their ability to frown, but even the activation of brain circuitry that hosts negative emotions (such as the amygdala) became less pronounced.[11-12] Researchers are next evaluating this approach to help patients with depression.[13-14] Fascinating!

Finally, several studies show that implementing self-affirmations can improve stress symptoms and cortisol levels,[15-16] anxiety,[17] physical health,[18] and medication compliance.[19] Among students with limited resources or low performance, self-affirmation has significantly decreased the performance gap.[20-21] Researchers are even finding activation of specific brain areas including the reward system and the self-referential regions of the brain with self-affirmation.[22]

Overall, affirmations have two goals: to heal our inner child and awaken our inner sage. A good affirmation is slightly nuanced so that it forces you to focus, engaging your attention. It must also be believable. Consider meditating on any of the lines below that capture some of the details I have shared. If you wish, write a short paragraph to elaborate on the words, answering what, why, and how (what is this concept, why is it important, and how do I go about accomplishing it).

- I am worthy of respect despite being wrong at times
- My failures inspire me to continue getting better
- The goodness I see in others shows the traits I admire that I wish to embody
- I want to succeed so I can help others
- Failures keep me humble which makes me stronger
- Despite my many imperfections, a part of me is sacred and pure
- There may be days I don't like my looks, but my soul is pure and indescribably beautiful
- What is right about me is overwhelmingly more than what is wrong
- Others' rejection of me will prompt me to love myself even more

Each of these thoughts and their related meditation is an act of self-compassion.

Imagery

Almost two decades ago, while I was at a zoo, a young girl fell into the lion's enclosure right before my eyes. None of the zookeepers were around at that time. Seeing her mother wailing and not seeing a lion nearby, I jumped to bring the little girl back. Right then, two lions came out of their den rushing toward me. With my heart pounding and lungs hyperventilating I picked up the girl and ran. As the lions were closing in, I woke up, panting. There was no zoo, no lions, and I wasn't the brave person I had played out to be. But my imagination had riled up my entire hypothalamus, pituitary, adrenals, and the sympathetic nervous system. Imagination can be as powerful as the real thing.

Just as your imagination can raise your adrenaline, it can also activate the central part of your parasympathetic system, your vagus nerve, bringing you to a calm state.[23-24] A vagus-mediated calmness tremendously helps with creative thinking and cognitive performance.[25-26]

Countless videos and programs on guided imagery are available to cater to almost any preference. Think about what environment you prefer: ocean, greenery, mountains, grasslands, floating above it all, on a cruise, or something else. Pick a program based on that preference, find a comfortable place, start deep breathing, and then take your brain through the experience of being in that environment by listening to the soothing voice of the narrator.

Several dozen studies show the benefit of imagery: for pain and anxiety in children,[27-28] improving attention,[29] decreasing food cravings,[30] improving fatigue and quality of life in patients with cancer,[31] enhancing physical activity,[32] improving fibromyalgia symptoms,[33] and even decreasing the cost of medical care.[34]

While imagery in some form has existed for thousands of years, recently, we have rediscovered an even more powerful form of imagery that truly transports you into a different world by creating a multidimensional virtual reality (VR). From a completely unknown intervention in the 1990s, hundreds of trials have now tested VR-based approaches for a wide variety of challenges. These include improving cognition and executive functions in seniors,[35] decreasing pain and generalized anxiety,[36-37] reducing depressive symptoms,[38] training to manage social anxiety,[39] improving balance,[40] and in several educational initiatives.[41]

Sustained calming imaginations can transform our biology. Not all of us have access to a walk in the orchards or can watch the sun setting into the ocean through our bedroom window. But we can take our imagination to those places. And that may be enough.

Self-talk

I follow a two-minute rule with my family, friends, patients, colleagues, and the larger world. For the first two minutes that I meet people, I practice radical acceptance. I don't try to "improve" them, through my words, actions, or thoughts. Instead, I strive to focus on what is right and admirable about them. I created this rule to overcome my disposition to find faults in others the moment I saw them. It was costing me relationships, because many in my world, including my family, started associating me with feeling bad about themselves.

But I didn't follow this rule with myself. My self-talk gathered the worst expressions I had heard from others about me and played it back in my lingo. Why could I do this so effortlessly? It was because, unlike others, I received no pushback from me. In the garb of protecting my present and improving my future, my Psyche dominated my Esse.

I also felt that harsh words were holding me to higher standards. In my effort to improve the future, I kept roiling my present. But when that future became my present, I got busy improving the future (or the future future!). I didn't like it but couldn't help it.

Here are a few perspectives I have used to redirect my self-talk, even as I remain a work in progress.

- Talk about a hopeful future instead of the discouraging past
- Think of people who appreciate you rather than those who denigrate you
- Keep your purpose front and center in your self-dialog
- Focus on your efforts rather than the outcome
- Focus on your intentions rather than emotions
- Remember your constraints, not just your failures
- Keep the child within you alive who is more innocent than guilty
- Never use words for yourself that you wouldn't accept from others and that you wouldn't be proud of if your children said them
- Instead of talking about what you did badly, talk about the good you can do

When I struggle with finding a few good words for myself, music is my refuge. Believable positive words written and sung by someone who may have spent several decades perfecting the art of writing and singing always uplift me.

Be a helper/healer, not a martyr: Set boundaries [42]

I was talking to a very conscientious manager in a reputable company. So, I was a bit surprised when she said, "My organization will take the last drop of my blood and sweat if I am willing to give it to them. I think they just about did." As a woman leader in a male-dominated field, she learned that the only way to run a marathon was to scale it through several hundred-meter sprints. She got exhausted before she had run a mile. Then, she learned about setting boundaries and saying no.

When you set a boundary, you put a psychological limit on your participation or agreement. Setting limits is particularly relevant now because of the boundary erosion created by networking technologies and social media.[43] The American Psychological Association defines a boundary "as a psychological demarcation that protects the integrity of an individual or group or helps the person or group set realistic limits on participation in a relationship or activity."[44]

Boundaries are the ropes around the masterpiece.[45] The Mona Lisa has been vandalized six times; many more wannabe vandals failed because of the boundaries. While a museum masterpiece may have a dollar value, you are priceless. You deserve to set boundaries so you can preserve yourself in your quest to serve others. Not setting any boundaries makes you swing like a pendulum between disengagement and martyrdom. The extremes of self vs. other focus confuse people.

Instead, have consistency to create trust. Balance your respect of yourself with your duty to others. Get over your FOSNO (Fear of Saying No).[46] Saying no when you must won't take away the right opportunities. People value you more when you balance self-preservation and self-growth with serving others. This is because they find you better self-regulated and more accountable to yourself, which is as important as accountability to others.[47]

A particularly helpful concept is setting emotional boundaries. Setting an emotional boundary means two things:

1. Allowing only a few close people, those you know who like and love you and whose values you admire, to influence your self-worth.
2. Planting guilt-free imperfections knowing that you have a finite number of hours in a day and can't be at two places at the same time. You are then okay with not fully engaging in certain roles. For instance, if your role as a professional, mom, spouse, sibling, daughter, friend, and neighbor is already taking 16 hours in a day, then you let go of being a perfect niece, coach, and volunteer.

Other practices

I like my oat milk with chocolate powder and honey. Without adding much volume, honey and chocolate powder transform the oat milk's flavor.

The following additional ideas are the chocolate powder and honey for my days.

Tiny moments of compassion

"You are so careless." We often berate our kids when they lose something and can't find it. Wandering around the house searching for a lost item can be a lonely depressing feeling. The rule at my home is that no one searches alone. If I see Sia searching for her school bag, I drop everything and join her. Now, she reciprocates the same, as does everyone else. Lending a compassionate hand when others feel vulnerable helps them feel comfortable sharing their vulnerabilities instead of hiding and stewing on them. Find such tiny moments of compassion for others. They will return the favor, if not today, certainly at a later date.

Micro-celebrations

Phenomenal success is phenomenally rare, but small wins happen all the time. A lot goes right for your mocha to taste like a mocha. You have buying capacity, live in a world willing to serve you, are not allergic to the ingredients, have sensitive taste buds, and appreciate the taste of coffee. Celebrate the simple that hides the profound. The work of a ceiling fan, the dancing leaves on the trees, the water in the faucet, the icemaker in your freezer, and all the people who create and upload great self-help videos are phenomenal luxuries worth celebrating. If you are willing to lower your threshold, you might have something to celebrate daily.

Body on mind

You might be surprised that one of the first positive effects of healthy nutrition and moderate exercise isn't improving our physical health. It is feeling more upbeat.[48-49]

Taking good care of ourselves keeps inflammatory chemicals (e.g., cytokines) in check, which helps with our fatigue, mood, and vitality. Similarly, making sure that the air filters at your home are not too old or clogged, the water you drink doesn't have undesirable impurities, the radon level in your home isn't high, and you are not consuming microplastics or heavy metals in your food all help your immune system and other body organs stay in top form so you can continue to do good in the world.

Posture

Experts differ on the value of the "power pose," with some studies supporting a mild effect on confidence and willingness to engage,[50-51] while other studies show a completely negative result.[52] Nevertheless, most people and experts agree that maintaining a good posture is important for personal health and well-being. But is there a universal good posture? Common sense tells us that it might be different for someone with a healthy spine compared to a person with chronic pain from a spinal condition. Thus, we presently do not have a scientifically proven universal definition of a good posture.[53-54]

With those caveats in mind, experts suggest gently maintaining the spinal curves, keeping the head aligned with the shoulders, the shoulders above the hips, and staying agile.[55-56] In simple words, be aware of your body, avoid slouching your back, do not walk or sit with a turtleneck, and keep moving.[57] In addition, while sitting, it is good practice to support your back, hips, and thighs, and while walking, pull your shoulders slightly back and tuck your stomach in.

Research shows a good upright sitting and walking posture can affect your stress response, energy level, and depressive symptoms.[58-60] Having said all that, I must confess that I find myself slouching all the time!

Click Likes

We like to like. We also like to be liked. The reason is simple. Liking and being liked both activate our brain's reward network.[61-62] Further, disagreeing and disliking activate the insula and other brain areas that create an unpleasant feeling.[63]

The one caveat is authenticity. Forcing yourself to like what you dislike activates the brain's pain areas. So, the two-part solution is simple. One, try to surround yourself with good people whose values you admire. Do not go for quantity; focus on quality. In my view, every negative person undoes the impact of several positive people.

Two, assume positive intent (API), to the extent you can, for the annoying aspects of good people. But only to a limit. If their thoughts, words, or actions transgress your values or trespass into your self-respect, you must set your boundary and excuse yourself or take a corrective action, whichever is appropriate.

What do I need?

If you want to test your patience, try to help an overstimulated nine-month-old baby sleep. They will fight tooth and nail. I can't fathom why they get so jittery when being a little calmer can help them get what they want. We adults aren't much better.

Often, we can't parse between our needs and wants. I won't belabor the difference between the two except for sharing a story. I once met a financially insecure gentleman to help with his fractured relationships and high levels of stress. He had over twenty million dollars in the bank, the same amount in retirement savings, and a sprawling real estate. Yet, he was insecure that he wouldn't have enough if something bad was to happen. He was also stuck in comparison traps because his friends had more. "I need at least double of what I have," he said.

He was confusing wants for needs. He needed contentment, purpose, a deeper engagement with the good people in his life he could trust, and the skills to be okay with some uncertainty.

When you feel antsy, often the cause is related to seeking or avoiding something. In those moments, consider answering the following: What is my primary need that isn't presently satisfied — is it the need to feel secure, to be respected, to be loved, to feel in control, to find a purpose, or something else?

A simple awareness of your needs can bring you peace. It can also help you direct your thought force toward more satisfying endeavors. There is no point chasing a specific number in the bank account if your primary need is to feel respected.

Potpourri

We will conclude this part with a potpourri of ideas for some of which the biological basis is still under research.

Grounding/Earthing

Some researchers believe that spending time in direct touch with the earth's surface can help the human body's physiological systems. Called Earthing, this contact might provide "electric nutrition" by transferring electrons to the body from the earth.[64-65] In several studies, researchers report a change in cytokine and white cell levels with a resulting decrease in inflammation and auto-immunity, and better wound healing.[66] A few studies have shown a decrease in blood viscosity,[67] increased physical energy, decreased mental stress,[68] lower pain,[69] and potential improvement in several diagnoses ranging from infectious diseases to neurodegenerative conditions.[70] While the science is still under development, I have started removing my socks once in a while when I can walk on clean nicely paved ground, free of rocks, bugs, and sharp stuff.

Gratitude journaling

Your dining experience at a restaurant depends less on the menu and more on what you order from the menu. Similarly, if you consider all the world's experiences as one extensive menu, then what you notice and focus on matters the most for your life's experience.[71-72] One way to improve your attention to what is going right in your life is through gratitude journaling.

Research shows several benefits of this simple discipline. These include improved depression and anxiety scores in health care workers,[73] improved burnout in pediatric residents,[74] enhanced academic motivation among university students,[75] lower inflammation and better asthma control,[76-77] and improved psychological distress and quality of life among patients with advanced cancer.[78] Consider giving gratitude journaling a try, particularly if you do not instinctively think grateful thoughts on many days.

The happiness of feeling grateful is distinct compared to the pleasure of savoring an ice cream. So, be grateful for the ice cream you are eating to double the joy!

Massage

Who could argue with a good massage?! Several dozen studies have proven the benefit of massage for chronic stress, anxiety, and pain.[79] Massage is a wonderfully relaxing, calming, and pleasing lifestyle intervention that, in the right hands, has minimal to no side effects and can improve overall well-being and even the health of the immune system.

Yoga

Hundreds of studies have evaluated the benefit of yoga for a wide variety of diagnoses, including back pain, carpal tunnel syndrome, asthma, diabetes, hypertension, irritable bowel syndrome, fibromyalgia, chronic stress, and several other medical conditions.[80] Yoga is also a valuable approach to maintaining optimal health. If you plan on practicing yoga, please take instructions from a trained teacher and start with gentle postures and breathing exercises that do not ask you to become a human pretzel.

Supplements

In people with clearly demonstrated deficiencies such as vitamin B12, vitamin D, or iron, supplements can have a remarkable effect on health and well-being. After studying the effect of subtle micronutrient deficiency on the health of our immune system and how common these deficiencies are, I feel compelled to increase my intake of foods that provide these nutrients. Let's save a more elaborate discussion of nutrition for another time.

Finally, avoid smoking and drug use, and minimize alcohol intake. Even one to two drinks daily are associated with a lower brain volume.[81]

Let's say you spent the whole day in a perfectly air-conditioned room with the ideal temperature, humidity, lighting, music, and aroma. You didn't sweat, and the creases on your clothes remained well preserved. Would you like to wear the same clothes after you take a shower the next morning? Probably not. No matter how perfect the atmosphere, our clothes and bodies get a bit dirty. The same is true about spending time with us and others.

Even if you are perfect, you and the world will likely find annoying aspects within you. Some of these you can improve right away, a few might take time, and a few are just how you are.

Fortunately, self-compassion is just one among many ways to find peace with oneself. The other two well-researched approaches are self-acceptance and self-forgiveness. Next, let's explore the theme of self-acceptance, which permits you to love yourself even as you strive to improve.

SELF-ACCEPTANCE

30
Eight Billion Sages

> Pick the title of your biography — suffering or overcoming. The chapters that fill the book will follow.

Self-acceptance and self-forgiveness are some of the more difficult practices that call for an even deeper insight into our nature. So, let's briefly revisit our Esse/Psyche model of the self, which will set the stage for accessing and healing a part of us that may be hurtful.

Archaic and modern

A seed isn't just a bead of fiber and nutrients. It carries intellect and an impulse to recreate its source. Books are more than a collection of cellulose sheets. Books are alive with words that can give you hope, bring you to tears, and connect you with someone who walked the earth two thousand years ago. You and I are not just skin bags packed with body organs. We are more than what the eyes can see. We embody thoughts and emotions that serve a purpose, share love, and for many, find strength from faith. Almost every entity has a higher-order reality. Our Esse, or any other name you wish to choose, is our higher-order reality.

We feel closer to our Esse when we are fully immersed in a meaningful task, or, for many, in deep prayer. Such experiences, which have an element of flow, purpose, and altruistic intention, are sadly but an oasis during a typical day. Most of our days are dominated by the drift of our ever-changing Psyche.

In addition to our conscious experiences, our Psyche, as I shared earlier, is a repository of repressed memories and emotions that we may or may not be able to recall (our subconscious and unconscious mind) yet that affect our present moment conscious experience. For many, these memories and experiences are of a traumatic past that deprived them of love and psychological safety.

Thus, while my Esse thinks of gratitude, kindness, and forgiveness, my Psyche thinks of survival, safety, and sustenance — two important yet different goals. In a tug-of-war between gratitude and survival, which priority would nature choose?

Psyche's survival and safety initiatives, however, are archaic. In evolutionary terms, just yesterday Psyche dominated Esse in fighting the Neanderthals. Imagine if our ancestors forgave men running at them with clubs and spears. We absolutely needed our Psyche to dominate then.

A lot has changed in the past few thousand years. Most present-day Neanderthals are emotional and symbolic, with many attacking us from inside our minds. Calling the entire fire department to douse a sparkler won't be a good use of resources. We would embarrass ourselves if we did that. But that's what our Psyche does — its reaction sometimes hurts more than the pain of the original insult.

Further, our repressed traumatic memories and emotions heal through wisdom and love, not by letting them dominate our minds and create a never-ending echo. The source of that wisdom and love within us is our Esse.

For healthy emotional well-being, we need to tap into our Esse and tame our Psyche, a striving that will continue challenging me for the rest of my life. That striving got a big boost several years ago when I met an enlightened teacher who happened to be a patient of mine.

My patient my teacher

Life sometimes offers experiences that change everything. For me, it was taking care of a thirty-year-old girl named Natalie. Natalie had a severe heart condition concurrent with kidney failure. She knew she only had a few more months. Her very advanced illness didn't meet the criteria for any curative therapy. Natalie couldn't lie down or complete sentences because of her shortness of breath. She wouldn't laugh because even a tiny giggle became a spasmodic cough.

Yet, Natalie, who had little time left, knew how to make the most of it. Stress moves you — the direction you get to choose. Natalie chose to move upward with stress. She didn't complain about the lack of medical options and wasn't angry with God. She mostly talked about love, forgiveness, and gratitude: how she overcame her fear with love, anger with forgiveness, and sadness with appreciation.

As a result, she was at perfect peace with life. In one of her ethereal moments, Natalie experienced the union of wisdom, love, and grace, in the light of which she saw her essential nature. "For once, the fog cleared, and I could see the light illuminating the darkest corners."

She felt a deeper presence that softened her insecure inner voice with compassion. "As if there are two "Natalies" within me," she said. "One is fearful of the curtain falling; the other is excited about what awaits me on the other side. Most days, I feel excited."

Natalie's experience paralleled the Esse and Psyche I have been sharing with you. Her Esse had tamed her Psyche. Every time I met her, I was uplifted. "What if we live our entire lives with love, forgiveness, gratitude, and compassion, much before we get an ultimate diagnosis?" I wondered after talking to her.

A few weeks later, Natalie's mother called me to share that she passed away peacefully in sleep. It has been over a decade, but her gravelly voice, perhaps from her thickened vocal cords, still echoes in my head at least once a week. Inspired by Natalie, I started searching for a more profound presence within me that would compassionately smile at my insecure Psyche.

Before that, I had read a lot about self-compassion. I had tried to be kind to myself for my inability to save the young man who was having a heart attack. I had tried to tell the mom whose emotional abuse contributed to her son's drug addiction, that parenting mistakes are common. I had comforted the girl who didn't pick up a phone call from her suicidal brother, nearly leading to the unimaginable. None of that made a huge impact. But now, helping people recognize that they still had a preserved purity within them despite their mistakes gave them hope. Knowing that you already have something that you just need to discover is much easier than treasure hunting without knowing what you seek. I recognize that not everyone is receptive or ready for such discussions. Still, in my experience, most find them helpful, immediately or with time, after they have assimilated our conversation and made it their own.

It is tough being human given that we didn't create ourselves. Sometimes, we overthink our happiness away. Given our propensity for self-blame, hurtful ruminations, and the load of worries we must lift, I try to live every day with Natalie's wisdom.

I share this wisdom with patients, particularly those carrying a haunting past or an insecure future. It gives them peace. A forty-year-old with stage four colon cancer once asked me, "This is so helpful and makes so much sense. Why didn't I think about it when I had more time five years ago?" I think our fear, desire, and ego stir up so much dust of ignorance that we can't see with clarity.

Friend, despite what the world tells you, no matter how much others disapprove of or despise you, you have a preserved pure core, your Esse. Even though something bad may have happened because of you, the core of you is still unblemished. Even though you might have experienced rejection from others, your Esse is phenomenally beautiful. Anchoring your identity in your Esse will dismantle the last shred of inner loneliness.

So, let your Esse empower you to tame your lower impulses, looking at your Psyche with compassion, acceptance, and forgiveness. You will find a path to self-love, and no matter how big or small your contribution, bring blessings to your world like a sage.

Brutes, self-serving, humans, sages

Watching an alligator viciously attack an innocent gazelle in water, I wondered how the alligator would hunt if he had the capacity for compassion. A very small proportion of humans are like an alligator, devoid of compassion. The primal instincts to eat, not get eaten, and reproduce drive their lives.

Visiting the Colosseum a year ago, I couldn't help but think about the 400,000 gladiators, prisoners, enslaved people, convicts, and millions of animals who died there because a few humans with infantile compassion hardware rose to rule the rest. Many of those rulers were the brutes.

Better than the brutes are many who we call self-serving people. They aren't necessarily cruel to others, but they don't care much about them either. They have the capacity for growing in wisdom and love, but their ignorance-fueled confidence and ego limit their possibilities. Many of them seek just personal fortunes and some become very successful at hoarding vast sums of resources. A few rise to become senior leaders, raising their pay packages while asking everyone else to exercise austerity. One such gentleman I met a few years ago was too leery to have happier employees. "They might lose their performance edge," he said. I looked the other way to roll my eyes.

At the next level, where most of humanity is presently, depending on the situation, the Esse or the Psyche predominates. A lot depends on the most recent experience, the presence of the right (or wrong) role models, and the current level of contentment. You may have seen the same person who donated vast sums to charity get indicted and imprisoned for insider trading.

Finally, among a select few, Psyche is just about enough to support their survival and safety, while Esse dominates their thoughts, words, and actions. Such people are the salt of the earth. They don't have to be formal preachers. They could be a nurse, a teacher, an engineer, a doctor, a janitor, a teller, an airline agent, an attorney, a police officer, an entrepreneur, or someone else.

During all known human history, we have had people in all four groups: brutes, self-serving, average humans, and sages. I strongly believe that with each passing century, collectively, our Esse is increasingly more expressed, and our Psyche is slowly receding in the background, having served its purpose (Figure 8). Eventually, I pray we reach a point where every person wakes up every day with just one identity — as an agent of service and love. That's when we will have eight billion sages on the earth.

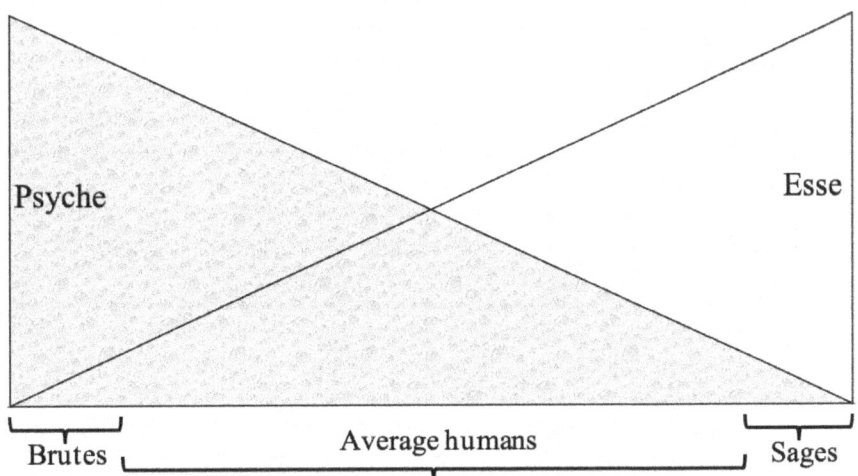

Figure 8. Evolution of the human mind

In that world, a formal practice of self-acceptance and self-forgiveness will likely not be needed since compassion will dominate our thinking. Until then, let's continue working on and with our imperfections.

31
What Is Self-Acceptance?

> A complete lack of fear, envy, and anger could be a sign of an unhealthy brain.

Acceptance is your willingness and ability to embrace the truth. In acceptance, you creatively work with what is, what was, and what might be. Acceptance stops fighting the wind so you can adjust the sail.

Willingness and ability don't mean you must like every aspect of the truth. Let's say after a 30-minute wait at a drive-thru, you get your lightly sweetened hot Latte in 2% milk with a squirt of hazelnut. As you drive out and take the first sip, it is black coffee with no sugar. You want to turn around, but the place is bustling, and you're in a hurry. What would be your response?

1. Call the coffee shop to take out your frustration
2. Stay upset for the rest of the drive
3. Instead of getting upset, feel grateful for a low-calorie drink
4. Get momentarily upset, but still give the drink a try

If you had asked me two decades ago, I may have responded with the first or second option. Now, I would pick the fourth. The third one is the best response, but for some, might be boringly idealistic. You want some drama in life, don't you?!

Acceptance helps you preserve your balance through life's natural turbulence so that you are predictably kind to others and yourself. An integral part of acceptance is accepting the self.

What is self-acceptance?

Self-acceptance is your willingness and ability to embrace all aspects of yourself. These include your physical being, thoughts, emotions, values, your actions, the work you do, and your spiritual beliefs. You could also include your relationships and possessions.

Here also, willingness and ability don't mean you have to like every aspect of you. Remember my youngest child (dog) Simba, who leaves small, smelly puddles on our floor in excitement?! I don't welcome them but given his job profile as the chief happiness officer of our home, he has so many other great qualities that I am happy to embrace this aspect of him, even as I continue to improve it.

Similarly, I would love to chisel my persona to carve a more symmetrical countenance. I wish I had a deeper voice, a better sense of humor, a higher pushup score, paid lower taxes, etc. At some point, however, I realized that in my effort to improve, I did not appreciate how good it already is. Further, with two-thirds of the earth covered in clouds, it's going to rain on my parade someday. That's only fair.

That awareness helps me remember to exhale deep and slow on most days. I am still a sophomore in the school of self-acceptance, but at least better than I was in my freshman year.

Finesse with self-acceptance involves four progressive components (ALiVE): Acknowledge, Let-in, Value, and Empathize.

Four components

A key isn't necessarily the most photogenic structure. But it does its job precisely because of that reason. Its beauty isn't in its smoothness or symmetry. The beauty is in how well its serrations match the lock it fits.

Similarly, every aspect of you has value in the proper context. If that value isn't seen or realized today, it is not because you are less capable. It is because you haven't yet found the right lock. Trust me, it is waiting for you. Given how small our world has become, it can't be too far.

With this conviction, let us look at the four **ALiVE** components of self-acceptance.

1. Acknowledge

Richa's mother endearingly called her *Bittu* at home, a name her friends found comical in elementary school. Once, her uncle came to her school for an early pick up. When the teacher called for *Bittu*, Richa didn't budge from her seat or recognize her uncle! She would rather stay at school all night than be a laughingstock by acknowledging her embarrassing nickname.

The first step to self-acceptance is acknowledging the parts of you that you would rather deny. Fortunately, the world has phenomenally changed in the last few decades. When you own up to your imperfect past, people give you a standing ovation. The reason is simple: people love to feel validated. Seeing your imperfections helps them feel worthy.[1-2] They find you relatable.

Assume you are the sky, and everything happening in life is the weather. You, the sky, remain untouched by the dry spell and the thunderstorm. Such an awareness might make it easier for you to acknowledge and eventually accept what you were earlier rejecting.

2. Let-in

When I first moved to the U.S., my English was decent, but my accent sometimes created frustrating moments. Imagine how fun it would've been to order a pizza on a cellphone with a bad connection. I had my share of pepperoni instead of bell pepper.

Fearing awkward moments, I avoided social gatherings, phone conversations, and small talk during daily life. Such avoidance behaviors provide temporary relief but seldom solve the problem.[3]

Soon, I realized my senior patients would crank up their hearing aids right when I started speaking. I felt embarrassed at having to repeat my words. Something had to be done. I found a temporary solution in writing or drawing my thoughts for my patients as I spoke. Every one of them went home with a couple of sheets.

My patients were very considerate and took it all in stride. Feeling validated, I let my accent be a part of me, even engaged in some self-deprecating humor. The newfound ease gave me the poise to start enunciating loud, clear, and slow. Eventually, I found a way to roll my r, simultaneously with taking the U.S. Citizenship oath!

3. Value

"You sound artificially intelligent, the way you speak," Dr. Brooks, one of my colleagues, said after a talk. I couldn't make out whether he was serious or poking fun at me. Nevertheless, I took him in stride. I started finding value in my oddities, letting them integrate into my persona. (If you ever watched my TEDx talk or any other video, please let me know if that is indeed true.)

Valuing differences is a key ingredient in self-acceptance. Once you take pride in your heritage, you start internally feeling that you belong. If all musical instruments sounded identical, you wouldn't have an orchestra. Thus, your voice has a unique value, just like any other.

Workplace belonging needs two key ingredients: the outside world embracing you for who you are, and you embracing yourself for who you are. Fostering employee self-acceptance is thus critical to nurturing a sense of belonging.

4. Empathize

Self-empathy opens your eyes to your struggles. Next time when you are socially isolating, lost in your thoughts, not speaking up at meetings, leaving parties too soon, or drinking excessively, recognize that all of these could be markers of denying or suppressing a part of the self.

Self-empathy, however, isn't easy. This is partly because, with self-empathy (like self-compassion), we feel we are lowering our standards and giving ourselves a free pass. How can we continue to improve while feeling content at the same time? Psychologists have a particular name for the conflicted state of our mind — dissonance.

Dissonance

The word dissonance is often used in music when two notes lack harmony. In daily life, cognitive dissonance happens when you must hold two conflicting thoughts (beliefs, values, attitudes) at the same time. The lack of congruence between our thoughts or between beliefs and actions is discomforting. The discomfort propels us to make a change in thoughts or actions to minimize the incongruence.[4]

The classic story is the fable of "The Fox and the Grapes." When the fox cannot get the grapes, to decrease his cognitive dissonance, he tells himself that the grapes are sour, so he no longer wants them.

Self-acceptance produces cognitive dissonance in a culture that values striving and growth. We are expected to work on our weaknesses, constantly improve, and challenge our assumptions. How does one grow if one is to accept one's imperfections?

In the discomfort of dissonance, we tend to preserve what we value more while compromising the conflicting thoughts or behaviors.[5] In a few cultures that value peace and acceptance over economy, industrial productivity and GDP growth lag, resulting sometimes in limited resources for subsistence. In the rest of the world dominated by a capitalistic drive, we flog ourselves, creating work-related cognitive and emotional overload that has pushed us on the brink of burnout.

With this state of our minds, the higher our GDP, the worse our mental health. That doesn't bode for a peaceful world since seldom does any country aim to stall its economic progress.

The question is, can we have our cake and eat it too? In other words, can we experience both self-acceptance and growth striving? Can we be a masterpiece yet a work in progress? I believe the answer is yes. Here is how I do it. It goes back to recognizing my Esse.

The two-part model

I accept the core of me, knowing my true essence is my Esse. Simultaneously, I let Psyche do the job of growth striving. I recognize my Psyche as an imperfect instrument, knowing that the repressed hurts within it will always keep it a work in progress. It will feel insecure at times, get greedy and selfish, and envy others. I do not judge it any more than I judge my Simba for going in circles chasing his tail.

With my Psyche, however, I do have one expectation. As I get older, wiser, and more content, I expect my Psyche to increasingly align with my Esse. I want my goals to become more altruistic. I want to earn so I can share, learn so I can help, and personally grow to nurture others.

I hope that with time, as my Psyche sheds its insecurities, it will progressively become like my Esse. I wouldn't have to try to be altruistic. Temptations would naturally stop supplanting higher values. The joy from compassion will replace my love for material gains. I will feel free.

32

Self-Acceptance: Why

—— ✦✦✦ ——

> Accepting the rain increases the joy of the sunshine.

Grades have tortured me all my life. In elementary school, I started at the higher end of the alphabet, D through F, unlike Richa, who had never seen anything below an A. As a sixth grader, she would have rejected me before a Hello. On one of my third-grade reports, I scored a three out of a hundred in math. "How did you score a three out of a hundred when most other kids with just a little effort scored above 80 percent?" Richa can never fathom it.

My rational first excuse to my parents was that someone must be at the bottom for others to be at the top. I was surprised when it fell flat. It seemed logical and well-articulated. Nevertheless, I tried a second argument. "I am training to go big in cricket. That's what smart boys do," I said.

It worked until one summer when my family visited my precocious cousin, who was quadruple accelerated, clean as a freak, and had started flossing at age 8 when I still didn't regularly brush my teeth at night. To top it all off, he was good at sports, too. Thankfully, in a few weeks, my parents forgot all about him, and I was back at the playground.

I am convinced that unless I made it big in cricket, which happens to 0.0001 percent of players, I would have been a street vendor in some unnamed corner. What saved me was developing a neurological illness. The episodes of passing out and the side effects of the medications took me off the playing field. With no access to video games or girls to date, fiction books became my respite. Non-fiction quickly followed, transforming (or degrading) me into a grade-obsessed bookworm.

With that came better exam scores, which brought the welcome attention and a bit of popularity. Eventually, the hamster forgot why it got on the wheel. But this hamster needed more depth and an anchor. His self-worth was as good as the next grade.

Eventually, when my academic bubble burst, older, deep-seated hurts resurfaced — that of early rejections, medical condition, envious words, and competition. I felt unworthy again, unhappy in my skin. The more I looked inward, the worse I felt. That's when I turned to reading philosophy and spiritually uplifting books, writing poems, and meditating. One day, seeing the moon with a good pair of binoculars gave me a useful insight.

The binocular effect

The moon is a gorgeous sight for your bare eyes. Look at it with binoculars, though, and you see countless scars.

That's what happened to me. The closer I looked at myself, the more scars I saw.

Thankfully, I took the moon metaphor further. Is it fair to judge the moon for its scars when billions of rocks pelted its surface creating the disfigurement? "Are my insecurities, fears, temptations, and guilts my fault, or are many of these related to external hurts?" I wondered. I invite you to ask yourself the same question.

That's the first why of self-acceptance. The second reason for self-acceptance is knowing how it can benefit you through many research studies. Although it might be evident to you, let me briefly share what the science tells us.

State of the mind

Our world's psychological troubles are growing much faster than many other challenges. When I was in college, mental fitness was considered a great asset but not essential for survival. That's no longer the case, particularly for our youth.

One out of three U.S. adults experienced a mental illness or substance use in 2022,[1] with the rate even higher among young adults (age 18 to 25).[2-3] In the U.S., one person dies every eleven minutes by suicide, with over 12 million people having contemplated that possibility.[4] Among adolescents, suicide is consistently one of the leading causes of death.[5]

Despite the high prevalence of mental disorders, only one out of two adults with a diagnosable mental condition can afford the treatment, and a shocking 93.5% of adults with substance use disorder did not receive any treatment in the previous year.[6]

These statistics represent only the diagnosed conditions. Equally sobering are the numbers around languishing, loneliness, low self-worth, violence, divorce, and child abuse. We are materially wealthy yet emotionally poor.

Providing high-quality psychological and psychiatric care is only part of the solution because that is a reactive approach and will only impact the tip of the iceberg. The proactive approach to building societal resilience and mental fitness through improving self-worth, self-compassion, self-acceptance, and self-forgiveness, helping people find and connect with their purpose, and organizing our world around relationships will address the depth of the iceberg. Add to that addressing the social determinants of health (environment, poverty, living conditions, education, and more).

Let's next review a few research studies around self-acceptance as a prelude to transitioning into skills.

Research on self-acceptance

Researchers have examined the correlations and impacts of deficits in self-acceptance in several groups and for different conditions. I'll briefly summarize some of their findings.

Impact of Adverse Childhood Experiences (ACE)

The harmful impact of ACE on health and well-being was partly mediated through ACE causing lower self-acceptance among children.[7]

Self-acceptance protects against the mental health deterioration that can happen with ACE.[8]

Teenagers

Low self-acceptance was associated with appearance-focused comparisons that, when excessive, hurt body image and mental health.[9-12]

Low self-acceptance and high social comparison were associated with higher anxiety and depression among adolescents.[13]

College students

Low self-acceptance was associated with higher social networking site usage and materialistic values.[14]

Low self-acceptance worsened loneliness feelings among college students with visual impairment.[15]

Adults

Individuals with low self-acceptance were more likely to experience post-traumatic stress disorder from intimate partner violence.[16]

In people with stutters, high self-acceptance correlated with less perceived discrimination, less hostility toward others, and more successful therapy outcomes.[17]

In a study of over 4000 adults, higher self-acceptance was associated with greater generativity (caring + extending self into the future).[18]

Nursing home residents with low self-acceptance experienced lower subjective well-being.[19]

Self-acceptance may enhance longevity by up to three years.[20]

My friend and colleague Daniel Schwartz, one of the world's "25 most influential philanthropists," founder member of The Commons Project, and former board chair of the GAVI campaign, shared the benefits of self-acceptance in a recent communication with me. In his words, "My own increasing self-acceptance has been accompanied by an increasing acceptance of others in my life, making it easier for me to recognize, with compassion, the intrinsic human dignity and inherent value of everyone else." I admire his work and totally resonate with his experience.

Many of the effects of low self-acceptance work through keeping your brain's emotion centers riled up. Acceptance, on the other hand, calms your limbic system.[21] Let's see how we can do that through actionable insights and specific practices.

33

Self-Acceptance: How (Insights)

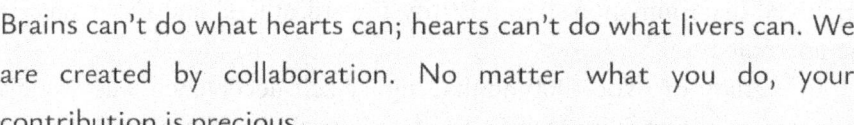

> Brains can't do what hearts can; hearts can't do what livers can. We are created by collaboration. No matter what you do, your contribution is precious.

A colleague who leads a large academic medical center grew up with a tough, dominant father who could never be pleased. She still feels unaccomplished despite a distinguished career spanning two decades.

A middle-aged C-suite executive received a surprise divorce notice in the mail after twenty years of marriage. With her ex now dating one of her friends with whom he has had a steady affair for the last two years, she feels cheated at every level. Despite being an amazingly compassionate person entrusted with multiple major responsibilities, she feels something is wrong with her, which is why people keep rejecting her.

A multimillionaire real estate developer seldom feels connected to anyone. "Everyone who meets me wants a part of my skin. I have no real friendships." He feels he is incapable of making friends.

A very successful manager with an amazing family has never grown out of the embarrassment of being only five feet three inches tall. "Most of my colleagues' kids are taller than me," he says. He tries to act macho to compensate for his height and baby face, sometimes running into disciplinary issues because of his behavior.

A neurosurgery colleague can't forget one surgery over a decade ago where his mistake led to an intra-operative stroke in a young patient. He feels guilty about harming his patient even though his performance is much superior to that of other surgeons in his department.

Having met nearly twenty thousand patients individually and several hundred thousand in groups, I could fill the following fifty pages with stories of people rejecting themselves. The vast majority are good, conscientious, competent people who narrow their focus on some part of their life that they can't accept. In the above examples, I intentionally shared stories of outwardly highly successful people who regularly experience self-rejection. Lack of self-acceptance is even higher among people with less storied lives.

In my experience, asking people to try blanket self-acceptance doesn't work. For no fault of theirs, for a long time they have allowed the not-so-good to dilute everything else that is wonderful, ending up rejecting the whole. This disposition becomes part of their identity that they cannot easily shed.

Below, I share some insights I have found helpful for myself, my patients, and my clients. Insights educate your mind that your efforts to forcibly push away your perceived imperfections lay a trap. This trap keeps you dueling with the self. A much better approach is to first limit your struggles to what is worth your time (values over preferences), look at (rather than look through) your thoughts, and be willing to experience the unpleasant.

Best not to confuse preferences for values

"I won't ever compromise my values." Sheila was talking to her husband about not letting her eighth grader drink any caffeinated beverage. Sheila didn't know that at every social opportunity, her daughter, because of the restrictions at home, was binging on coke.

Sometimes, we become inflexible about our preferences, calling them our values. We hold ourselves and others to unreasonable "standards" — won't ever have a drink with high fructose corn syrup, won't buy any product with artificial colorings, or refuse to take any pills that are round and white (I had one patient who was stuck with this preference). If we break this standard, we mistakenly reject ourselves — a common outcome of psychological inflexibility.[1]

I have a simple guiding rule: be flexible about preferences and strong in principles. Be firm about integrity, compassion, and commitments made, but for most of the stuff that won't matter in five years, go with the flow.

Do not flee the bear

"Do not run away from the bear," forest rangers say, "because then the bear sees you as a prey." You won't go far anyway, because the bear can easily reach a top speed of 35 mph.

The same holds true for fleeing a negative thought about the self. You can't outrun it. Fighting or playing ignorant won't work, either. The best approach is to look at it for what it is — just a chemical reaction among your brain's neurons.

The problem occurs when your Psyche fuses with the thought. Then, instead of looking at the thought, you look through it. The thought colors and distorts your world view.

Instead of letting that happen, consider placing your attention deeper than your thoughts, in your Esse. Look at your thoughts as external to you. Then smile at your thoughts like you might smile at a two-year-old throwing a benign tantrum. Just looking at thoughts instead of looking through them and recognizing that you are deeper than your thoughts might be enough to start freeing your mind from your thoughts' grip.

Like a negative thought, a repressed memory of a previous hurt is a neuronal network firing intermittently. Feeling compassion for the innocent you who had to endure the experience that created the storehouse of these thoughts will help you heal and progress in self-acceptance.

Willingness

One of my mentees had received twelve job interviews. He couldn't secure a job after the first eleven. The final interview was now very critical. Amidst intense preparations, he sought my help.

My suggestion was opposite to his plans. "Go there to fail," I suggested. "Meet your interviewers like they are your old college buddies. Negotiate a bit instead of agreeing to everything." The plan worked. His willingness to fail calmed his nerves, which helped him perform better than usual, getting him the job.

Your willingness to be imperfect makes you less imperfect. Be okay with your lack of singing talent, receding hairline, less-than-white teeth, or clumsiness with chopsticks. Your willingness to accept yourself as you are will free your energy to focus on what truly matters. You will manifest your Esse through your being. That's where your true beauty resides.

Language of hope

When you want to implement a change, instead of rejecting the present self, focus your thoughts and language on embracing the future self.

Which of the following two self-dialogs will inspire you more?

I hate my writing skills, or
I look forward to becoming a better writer.

I'm sure you like the second one better. Prioritize learning over worrying about others' judgments or judging yourself.[2]

Consider saying, "I can't wait to restyle my hair," instead of "I look worse than a porcupine." While the implication might be the same (not literally with the porcupine example!), words of future self-approval create better self-worth than words of present self-rejection.

Get comfortable with dissonance

Earlier, I talked about how cognitive dissonance creates conflicts in our heads that we resolve by preserving what we value more and letting go of the conflicting thoughts. Here is a combination of two conflicting thoughts: I am a good person, and bad things happen to me.

Understandably, many of us believe that good things should happen to good people. Children stuck with rough caregivers can't reconcile why, despite doing nothing wrong, they experience abuse at the hands of adults who should be loving them. When trapped in the conflict between their positive self-view and objective cruelty at the hands of the world, they reject the former. They start assuming they are a bad person and deserving of all their pain. That gives birth to a lifetime of shame proneness.

I have found a way out of this conundrum. That good things should always happen to good people would be true in a perfect world. But in an imperfect world, these rules don't apply.

The human world created by our minds indeed isn't perfect. Understanding and internalizing this truth is wisdom. It helps you accept that even for phenomenal people like you, bad things can happen without any fault of yours.

How about numbing?

Anesthesia works like a miracle, letting surgeons painlessly probe into the body's deepest recesses. But every anesthesia eventually wears off, leaving pain receptors bare and ready for action.

Thus, suppressing the emotional pain through numbing with chemicals that alter our minds isn't a sustainable solution. Opposite to that, it becomes a problem. Here is why.

Just as antibiotics for pneumonia must be stronger than the bug causing the illness, the numbing agent must be more potent than what is causing the pain. Eventually, the numbing agent takes over the brain, making the brain obsessed with repeating the dose, which then escalates into an addiction. This is the reason a lack of self-acceptance is an important underlying predisposition to many addictions.[3]

What's better than numbing is many of the self-acceptance practices I share next.

One of my co-presenters at the World Happiness Summit (WOHASU) was Professor Lord Richard Layard, co-editor of the World Happiness Report. He is amazing at capturing wisdom in short, pithy words. After the summit, as a respected senior leader of the well-being movement, when I asked him to share his insights on self-worth and self-love, he put it simply as, "Unconditionally accept yourself and others, for peace and happiness." That pretty much sums up the insights!

34

Self-Acceptance: How (Practices)

> Smile with your eyes as you unlock your phone. It will give you a thousand extra smiles every year.

One of the most stressful times for teachers is orientation day. New students bring personalities and backgrounds that aren't in teachers' control. Parents have lots of questions — about the curriculum, class size, social and emotional programming, how to challenge their child, methods of engagement, measures of academic progress, etc. Most are reasonable, but in every class, a few demand more attention than the teachers can give.

A few weeks before her school start date, I met Brenda, an elementary school teacher who participated in the SMART (Stress Management and Resiliency Training) program for public school teachers. "I feel judged by every parent," Brenda said. "The more anxious ones get on my nerves. This time of the year my blood pressure is always through the roof."

"What are you worried about?" I asked Brenda.

"That they will judge me. I don't want them to think I am not good enough for their child."

"But I have never felt that way about my kid's teachers," I said, and I fully meant it. "As a parent, instead of judging you, I want you to like me and my child."

That was an "Aha" moment for Brenda. Her task was not to try and impress the students and parents. It was to help them feel comfortable and liked. She didn't have to be perfect, just kind and responsive.

That year, Brenda focused on helping families feel comfortable instead of avoiding being judged. She accepted that she might not have all the details, and that's okay. A few weeks later, Brenda sent me a note saying that it was the least stressful, most enjoyable, and most effective orientation day she had ever had.

Confused Sapiens

Worker honeybees know what to do to succeed in this world. So do zebras, rhinos, lions, and all other animals, except humans. We change jobs an average of twelve times in our lifetime. Yet, despite putting in forty or more years at work, we struggle with purpose.

We aren't much clearer about our relationships either. Some very sad words I once heard during a consult were, "I divorced the woman I loved." We throw away loving relationships while hanging on to toxic ones for too long.

Many of our past actions that seemed perfect play out differently than planned. The guy who discovered Freon was celebrated in 1928 when we didn't bother about climate change. But now we blame him for punching big holes in our ozone layer.

Knowing that we all are a little ignorant about many aspects of life, think about why you struggle with self-acceptance. Is any aspect that you disapprove of unique to you? Or is it part of the human condition? Also, are there times when you aren't clear what is the best path for the long term?

Consider accepting yourself, knowing that almost everything you see wrong about you is probably correct from a different, kinder, and more authentic perspective. Also, countless factors beyond your knowledge or control shape who you are today. How can you then blame yourself?

Research also confirms this. When you improve your self-knowledge and self-feeling, you become more accepting of yourself.[1]

Language of validation

The first time our romantic partner says, "I love you," the words sound magical. With time, those words don't lose value, but they certainly lose novelty.

Many of us crave the words, "I respect you," from life partners, children, and work colleagues. Respect is the new language of love. Words that show respect are the words that validate.

Speaking the language of validation is simple. I use active voice when taking credit and passive voice when feeling blameworthy!

Remember Ronaldo, the opera performer who found his confidence back? Like him, I now believe in those who believe in me. I look at myself with the eyes of those who love and trust me unconditionally. You are who your dog thinks you are.

Instead of saying I failed or could have done better, I tell myself I gave it my best, and there will be a next time.

Allow yourself to be happy in honor of those who want you to be happy.

That comparison thing again

In one of the acceptance assignments, I asked my students to identify one or two annoying traits of someone close to them and then state why they were willing to accept them. Ralph, a very articulate hospital chaplain, talked about his wife. "She isn't the best at time management and sometimes haggles more than I like. But her integrity, love, compassion, faith — they are all impeccable. She is amazing about everything time cannot destroy."

Our instinct is to compare our weaknesses with others' strengths and their weaknesses with our strengths. This creates judgment toward others and low self-worth. Remember that every person is strong in his or her unique way.

So, if you must compare, then focus on the important thing, not everything. Focus on love and virtues instead of competition and appearance.[2] Do not be dispirited by material injustice. Because at the material level, the world, by design, is unjust.

When I look at the plight of children caught in war-torn neighborhoods, I feel guilty about my comfort. On the other hand, I might feel envious driving through some of the elite beach-front neighborhoods where an average home costs north of $25 million. Both are unhelpful, particularly the envy. It is best to feel compassionate for those struggling and inspired to do good in the world if nature gives you more resources. From that perspective, it is best to consider the assets we own as not ours but leased to us for a short time. They are ours to do good in the world, not store in a hidden offshore account.

As I read in an inspiring devotional: Every time you lend a helping hand, you make deposits in the treasury of the Divine.

Look at, not through thoughts

You know the waves because you know the ocean. The ocean is real, the waves but a transient surface undulation. The depths are unaffected by the waves, small or furious. Thoughts are the same. They are transient mind waves, while deep within, your Esse is unaffected by them. Anchor in your Esse to look at rather than look through your thoughts.

Just as the breath slows down when you start noticing it, thoughts slow down when you start noticing them. The slowing may provide you the space to get deeper. Your thoughts now become part of your environment. You can start playing with your thoughts, particularly the negative ones, from that deeper place.

Repeat the negative thoughts in a singing voice or a child's voice to decrease their seriousness. Or if you wish to stay serious, ask yourself, "Is this true? Do I know for sure this is true?" If not, then consider letting it go.

A perpetual company of our thoughts with a proclivity to believe them, particularly the negative ones, pushes away self-acceptance. Being able to distance from the thoughts and see them objectively, thus not buying into their every message, is a massive step toward accepting the Psyche.

You reach a point where you smile at your Psyche when it starts the drama. "There you go again, my dear Psyche! Thank you for trying to keep me safe and amused. I love you too!"

Freedom from others

Throughout most of my school and college years, I was averse to social connections. As an idealistic simpleton who was an easy target for rowdy colleagues, I felt anxious before meeting people and came out bruised from most gatherings. My healing journey has gone through four phases.

Phase 1: Avoidance – In this phase, my constant companion was my books. I seldom interacted with people and limited those interactions to formal greetings or academic conversations. This phase lasted about 15 years.

Phase II: Not troubled – Through my medical training, I had to connect with patients and their families who needed my care and compassion. I became comfortable in this role, but outside those confines, was still sensitive and vulnerable.

Phase III: Resilient – Gradually, as I developed better self-worth and embraced myself as I was, I became resilient to others' stares. I made a list of people who I knew cared about me. They were the only ones who I let influence my self-worth. For others, I became stoic and unemotional. I took their praise but rejected their critiques, other than learning from the critiques. This phase lasted until age 45.

Phase IV: Healing – Through understanding neuroscience and psychology, developing resilience programs, and learning from tens of thousands of patients, students, and clients, I try to see every person as special and struggling. With that awareness, instead of feeling judged, I send them a silent good wish. I try to embody a healing presence no matter where I am.

Presently, I toggle between II, III, and IV, but with each passing year I spend more time in IV. I must add that by no means am I proposing any expectations for your social connections because each of us has our own social appetite and level of comfort.

Nevertheless, for self-acceptance to be enduring and for you to enjoy social connections, it helps to progress toward accepting, loving, and healing others.

Here is the most important fact I know about relationships: <u>I love you when I love myself in your presence</u>. When you help others feel worthy, they will help you feel worthy, putting you both in a phenomenal upward spiral of life.

Do something nice

Esse and Psyche collaboratively generate your roles and values.[3] Roles are what you do, and values are what you consider important. When your values support your roles, and together, they help you feel you are a good moral person, you have a positive concept of the self.[4]

Many of us lack a positive self-concept that improves mental health and academic performance and supports behavior change.[5] This is because of conflicting roles or conflicts between values and roles.

For instance, as a person who believes in an egalitarian world, I feel guilty about living in greater comfort and safety while many live in abject poverty. However, my self-deprivation won't help anyone. A greater flexibility can come in handy here. It means I can compensate for my lack of performance in one domain with positive actions in another. Thus, when I am privileged to do something for those who can't pay me back in kind, I am at least partly repaying for living in relative comfort.

Given that we all are guilty of one or another infraction against Mother Earth or our fellow beings, most people I meet struggle with self-acceptance. Most weeks, do something, however small, to help fellow beings or the planet with nothing expected in return. Such actions are a great way to enhance self-acceptance. As entrepreneur and philanthropist Anu Jain said to me, "Happiest people are those who do for others."

Imagine something nice

What is more powerful, the receding horizon in the rearview mirror or the upcoming vistas in the windshield? Most argue that we learn from the past to live for the future.[6] Thus, thinking positively of the future compared to ruminating over the past causes much more brain activation in areas that host personally relevant and emotionally positive information.[7] These areas include the medial prefrontal cortex and the ventral striatum.[8] As a result, thinking about a hopeful future enhances psychological well-being and goal planning. That's why scientists have another name for humans — Homo prospectus.[9]

Several studies show that simply writing a short essay about your values decreases performance stress, thereby improving outcomes in a real-world scenario.[10-12] Writing an essay about our values makes us believe that we are likely to live by them, making us happier and more self-accepting.

Consider completing one of the following sentences (limit to just one for now). After writing, think about your specific actions and imagine how they might feel.
- One person I will go the extra mile to help this week is:
- My guiding value for tomorrow will be:
- A personal challenge I commit to overcome this week is:
- The one annoyance of my closest loved one I commit to accept is:
- I promise to work on the following life limiter this week (check one):
    o Prolonged sitting
    o Excessive fatigue
    o Emotional suppression
    o Hopelessness
    o Loneliness
- One personal value I will study more this week is:

When you engage yourself fully in this exercise, you might notice that just thinking about doing something positive might enhance your positive feelings about yourself. Let's see how you feel after fulfilling your promise!

Cheerleading to self-acceptance

Self-rejection, with its downstream negative mental health impact, spares no one. Miss USA, famous actors, brilliant comedians, gospel singers, rappers, Olympic winners, soccer players, professional wrestlers, celebrity chefs, fashion designers, country presidents, ruling royalty, career politicians, spiritual gurus — these accomplished figures and many more have died by suicide.

Despite years of working on emotional resilience, I know I am vulnerable to social anxiety and am always on the lookout for early warning signs. One of the ways I help thwart negative mental symptoms is through cheerleading myself — about the past, the present, or the future.

I expand my domains of self-acceptance by including values beyond the traditional measures of success.[13] I also shrink my self-rejection domains by minimizing contingencies to my self-worth. For example, older age is revered and associated with wisdom in many cultures, but not considered so positive in others.[14] So, as I'm getting older, I'm increasingly connecting age with wisdom and not osteoarthritis. Consider probing one or more ideas noted below to cheerlead yourself.

- One of my best memories of helping someone is:
- I am a unique blend of:
- The best compliment I have ever received is:
- I am proud of overcoming:
- I was hilarious when:
- I am proud of my:
- My patience came in handy when:
- My ability to forgive has helped my relationship with:

Every time you complete a line with humility and not haughtiness, you accept yourself a little more.

Peel the onion

The protective chemicals in onions (mainly syn-propanethial-s-oxide) irritate your tear glands, making you cry. These emotionless tears have a different chemical constitution than those from experiences touching you at a deep place within you — peeling another type of onion.[15] Here is a suggested sequence for a contemplative practice that has an element of acceptance.

1. Sit in a comfortable position, taking deep breaths with a longer exhalation.
2. Take your awareness deep in your physical body (try to access and place your attention at the center of your heart). Stay there for a minute.
3. Next, try to go even deeper, past your body and your thoughts — assume you are more profound than your desires, fears, and ego. Stay there for a few minutes.
4. Now, see yourself as a newborn, a child of life, unconditionally loved by nature.
5. Stay with that awareness for as long as you wish.
6. Gradually move back — to your mind, your physical body, and then the world around you.

In an interesting study involving over 200 people, remembered parental acceptance was associated with a greater adult self-acceptance.[16] I recognize that not every person may have received parental acceptance, and if you are one of them, think of someone else who may have unconditionally accepted you, including a higher being to whom you pray.

Avoiding avoidance

Despising the undesirable hurts you by making you weaker and foggy headed. The more you try to avoid an experience, the stronger its hold on you. Here are four approaches that can help you face your demons, improving your self-acceptance.

Proactively empower yourself: So much in life is about timing. After a patient sustains cardiac arrest, physicians have just a few minutes to revive them. Saving a drowning victim needs expeditious and skilled action. So does managing negative emotions.

Persistent negative emotions produce excess harmful neurotransmitters and hormones (like adrenaline and cortisol) that paralyze the brain's rational system. By the time these systems recover, a lot of damage may have been done.

That's why consider proactively empowering yourself with insights and skills in stress management, reframing, and active coping. Create a gratitude groove and a compassion nook in your brain that you can visit to renew yourself. Start today even if everything is going well for you so these places are available during moments of challenge.[17]

Become aware: Recognize your tendency to avoid discomfort, noticing how it provides temporary soothing but perpetuates the problem. Initially, you don't have to do anything more than labeling. Research shows that just becoming aware of and labeling an emotion decreases activity in the amygdala, the brain area that hosts negative emotions.[18]

Take a step toward, however small: For decades, I had buried the memory of the hospital night when I lost a young patient who I believe I could have saved. Perhaps, the fear of happening that again guided me away from becoming a cardiologist. Slowly, however, I have allowed my mind to visit that moment. I have become comfortable talking about it. It has led me to self-acceptance.

Recognize that your self-acceptance journey might progress at a snail's pace and that's okay. A forceful acceleration risks injury and fresh wounds from which it might take even greater effort and time to recover. If the going gets tough, use the balm of compassion and forgiveness to help with acceptance.

Know that the process might hurt: For the first year after I came to the U.S., I had to repeat much of my overseas medical training. I was supervised by students three years younger than me. Yes, it hurt my ego, but I swallowed my pride, taking it as a necessary part of the process. When my supervisor asked me how I was handling it, I owned up to my pain and shared something I had heard growing up: "To fortunes I sail, passing through narrow lanes!"

Deep within our body sits an important digestive gland, our pancreas. The pancreas produces enough enzymes to auto-digest our entire physical body. Nature has done a beautiful job of keeping the enzymes contained and only releasing enough amounts at the right place to digest the food.

Similarly, annoying and unwelcome parts of our past and present can become helpful when prevented from spilling over. One of the skills that helps us mop up the spill is self-forgiveness, our final ingredient of self-love.

SELF-FORGIVENESS

35
This You Know Already

> Forgive yourself, if you do not have a PhD in human relations or life's struggles.

Forgiveness doesn't mean justifying, condoning, excusing, or denying others' mistakes. Instead, it is intentionally letting go of hurts even though you were wronged. By forgiving, you choose to live your life in freedom based on your values. Very likely, you know a lot about forgiveness already, some of which I will recap here.

A recap of forgiveness insights

Forgiveness is for you. By forgiving, you disempower the other person from having an enduring effect on you. You give yourself freedom. You do not let someone who shouldn't be in the story of your life write the title of your story. Further, implementing forgiveness saves you time for gratitude and compassion. Forgiving someone at work might improve your relationships at home; forgiving someone at home might improve your performance at work.

Revenge feels transiently pleasing. In our brain, contemplating revenge activates the reward network. This makes forgiveness difficult since it goes against our basic survival instinct and desire for pleasure.[1]

Forgiveness is a process. Soon after forgiving, you are likely to forget that you have forgiven. You will need several reminders. Forgiveness is often a slow process, not an event.

Good luck with receiving an apology. Postponing forgiveness until you receive a formal apology could be a very long wait. Those who have wronged you are often unlikely to own up to their mistakes.

Forgiveness goes to the undeserving. Not uncommonly, the recipient of your forgiveness won't deserve your kindness. They may show no remorse. You may have let go of the expectation that they will ever apologize.

Pick only the battles that are worthy of your time. You can wake someone asleep, but not the person pretending to be sleeping. It helps to keep in mind that you are forgiving, so you do not give them the power to increase your risk of heart attack, stroke, and dementia.

Remove intentionality when you can. Forgiveness becomes much easier if, in your mind, you can find a way to remove intentionality from the other person's words or actions. Maybe they didn't know something or were acting out of a constraint or fear that they couldn't share with you. This isn't easy or simple because people most likely to hurt us are the ones most entrusted to love.

Take good care of yourself. You do not have to forgive someone who is likely to hurt you again. Forgiveness doesn't mean you won't protect yourself from future hurts. Forgiveness also doesn't mean you won't take the appropriate recourse, such as a legal action (if that's what the situation warrants).

Intergenerational trauma

You have probably heard stories about how inter-tribal animosity can continue for generations. Even today, countries or a coalition of nations continue to harbor animosity against others for centuries with no signs of letting up. They continue deploying precious resources for war that, used elsewhere, could educate, empower, and uplift their citizens.

How does that happen? Why don't a few wise leaders seek and enforce an enduring peace?

The sad reason is simple and understandable. We get caught in the folds of the revenge loop. The primary feeder into this loop is our inability to connect others' unacceptable behavior with our original infraction. Here is how it works (Figure 9):

1. For reasons best known to them, A attacks B.
2. B has no choice but to take revenge because not taking revenge will show weakness inviting future attacks.
3-4. A feels the revenge isn't justified or is disproportionate to A's original insult. As a result, A retaliates.
5. B, to protect themselves and show strength, counter-retaliates.

The process keeps repeating until one of the parties is remarkably weakened or eliminated, or in some instances, rationality prevails, and peace is re-established.

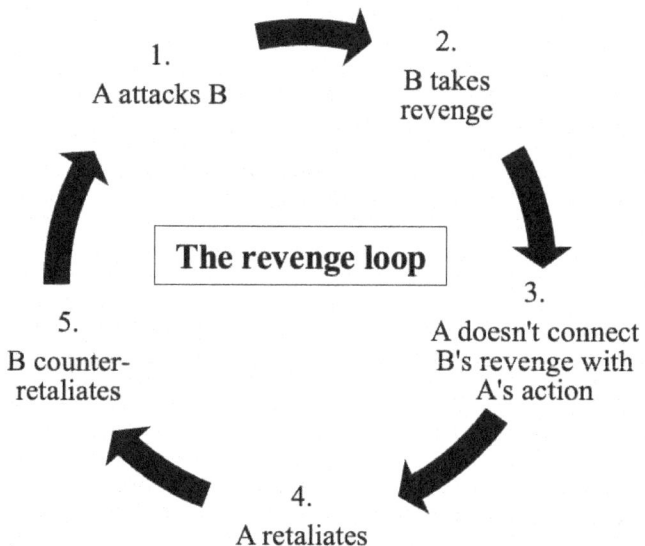

Figure 9. The circle of revenge

For both parties, retaliation seems reasonable because it sends a message that I am not an easy prey who you can attack without consequences. However, the retaliation instinct incurs a heavy cost. It converts a single indiscrete action into ongoing animosity for generations.

Revenge made sense for our ancestors, who were surrounded by robbers and pirates who burned their villages, looted property, and harmed the vulnerable. Forgiveness was construed as weakness, sometimes encouraging repeat insults. We believe in similar justice for criminals in current times. But revenge with a supervisor who did not recommend you for promotion or a driver who cut across the road may not be a wise choice.

This choice isn't wise also because the desire for revenge might fester within you for a long time, inflaming your system. Whenever you think of revenge, you give others a free pass to hurt you from the inside again. Why would you want to give anyone the power to repeatedly hurt you or cause you a chronic illness?

Opposite to revenge, the freeing practice of forgiveness has many benefits.

Benefits of forgiveness

While the precise neural mechanisms of forgiveness are still investigational, the most profound effect of forgiveness is on our cardiovascular and mental health.[2-4]

Researchers have looked at the benefits of forgiveness on mental health in several ways. Thus, correlative studies show that forgiveness is associated with lower depression, anxiety, stress, and aggression.[5] A large review of data from over 26,000 participants showed the positive effect of forgiveness on myriad mental health measures.[6] In a longitudinal study, a change in daily levels of forgiveness was associated with predictable change in stress and mental health symptoms over five weeks.[7] In a different design, researchers looked at the impact of lifetime stress on physical and mental health and found forgiveness was protective of stress-induced damage.[8]

Among physical conditions, forgiveness has the most demonstrable benefit on cardiovascular health indicators.[9] By calming our sympathetic nervous system, forgiveness helps with high blood pressure and lowers the risk of heart disease.[10] In an interesting study among patients with coronary artery disease, the effect of anger recall on decreased blood flow into the heart muscle was much less likely after learning and practicing forgiveness.[11]

Patients with chronic pain are another group that benefits from forgiveness. For instance, patients with fibromyalgia who experienced childhood abuse experience significant symptom relief with a forgiveness intervention.[12]

In a separate study, researchers found improved coping among patients with diabetes.[13]

An analysis of 128 studies (over 58,000 participants) showed that forgiveness of others was modestly associated with overall improved physical health.[14]

Increasingly, researchers are beginning to see forgiveness as a therapy for people with chronic medical conditions, many of which are strongly associated with early life adversity.[15]

Employers concerned with healthcare costs are also beginning to recognize the benefits of forgiveness. For example, in a workplace study of 108 employees, forgiveness was associated with better productivity and physical and mental health.[16] Another workplace study showed forgiveness was associated with higher job satisfaction, workplace engagement, and lower burnout.[17] With forgiveness also showing an association with better executive functions, I believe we have barely explored the benefit of this essentially free strategy to decrease healthcare costs, improve workplace metrics, and foster overall well-being.[18]

You might be curious if the benefits of forgiving others also apply to self-forgiveness. Even before that, what exactly is forgiving the self? Like self-compassion, self-forgiveness is sometimes confused with giving oneself a free pass. Let's clarify some misconceptions as we discuss the benefits of self-forgiveness and explore the path that takes us there.

36

The Five Steps

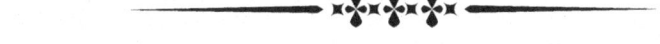

> When you try your best to be right, you earn a right to be wrong, and to be forgiven — by others and yourself.

Brad, a 52-year-old farmer and a dad of two teenage girls, was diagnosed with advanced prostate cancer. Brad hadn't visited a doctor in twenty years until an unremitting back pain led to an MRI and then the diagnosis. He had no family history of cancer, or so he thought, since he was adopted and didn't know anything about his parents. When his medical team made the effort to track down his ancestry, they found that several male members of his family had early-age cancers.

"If I knew my family history, I would have surely tested myself," Brad shared. He felt guilty. "Because of my negligence, my wife will have to raise my daughters alone." The self-blame, the regrets, the sorrow, and the fear pushed Brad into a downward emotional spiral.

Brad isn't the only one experiencing this. So is Eduardo, who blames himself for not insisting his nephew put on the seat belt, Ali, who regrets not speaking up when he first learned how his company was compromising on safety, Alex, for picking an unscrupulous financial advisor who led him to economic ruin, and Marianne, who wishes she could go back in time and say no to her daughter's sleepover. Good people are very good at feeling guilty with or without fault.[1]

The desire to change the past, the toxic guilt, the regrets, the self-blame — may all seem rational. But they are unhelpful. In excess, these feelings hamper rational thinking and prevent learning. A much better option is self-forgiveness.

Self-forgiveness: The basis

In high school, I got a bronze medal in an athletic competition. The caveat is that we only had three competitors! I didn't quite enjoy the award. Truth and fairness are essential for you to enjoy your success. The same is true for self-forgiveness. You won't truly benefit unless you feel you have earned it.

Self-forgiveness isn't self-excusing, self-blaming, self-punishing, or self-exoneration. It is intentionally letting go of resentment and letting in compassion that is anchored in owning up to mistakes, learning from them, and committing to making better choices in the future. Forgiving others doesn't have all these requirements since you can't force others to change, let alone expect them to feel guilty for what they said or did.

The dual process self-forgiveness model calls for reorientation toward positive values (accepting responsibility + making amends) and restoration of personal esteem.[2] While forgiving others is predominantly driven by self-compassion, authentic self-forgiveness needs a combination of compassion for others and compassion for oneself.

Like forgiving others, self-forgiveness doesn't mean you deny the wrong or close your eyes to the truth. It is recognizing that you are human. Self-forgiveness honors your constraints, trusts your intentions, and treats yourself kindly. It invites you to rethink your past more rationally and with greater compassion.

I asked my fellow WOHASU presenter, Professor Fred Luskin, director of the Stanford University Forgiveness Project and one of the world's pre-eminent forgiveness researchers, to summarize self-forgiveness for me. Here are his wise words: "Self-forgiveness is more of a behavioral than an affective process and must be earned rather than just felt. The ingredients are the honest expression of wrongdoing or mistakes, true remorse, making amends, and offering a sincere apology. When this process has occurred, one is free to let oneself off the hook and release any feelings of guilt or shame. It is more important to do good than to feel bad."

With that background, let's examine the research evidence supporting self-forgiveness before exploring the five steps that might help us on the journey.

Does it work?

The short answer is — yes! Research on self-forgiveness is almost as robust and equally (if not more) promising as research on forgiving others.[3] Below are some of the studies where researchers have reported that self-forgiveness helped.

- Decreasing problem drinking.[4]
- Improving physical health among college students.[5]
- Decreasing inter-generational transmission of adverse childhood experiences (ACE).[6]
- Staying resilient after abuse.[7]
- Maintaining psychological well-being and reducing psychological distress.[8]
- Decreasing suicidal ideation.[9]
- Lowering negative emotions in suicide loss survivors.[10]
- Decreasing risk of self-harm.[11]
- Lowering risk of self-injury among adolescents.[12]
- Lessening shame proneness.[13-14]
- Diminishing catastrophizing and negative emotions and enhancing active coping in patients with fibromyalgia.[15]
- Lowering rumination and improving sleep quality.[16-17]
- Increasing hopeful feelings.[18]
- Lowering the risk of cognitive impairment, particularly in people high on hostility.[19]
- Enhancing psychological safety among nurses.[20]
- Improving compassionate and balanced thinking about the self.[21]
- Enhancing overall health and mental health.[22]

All of these benefits accrue for almost no cost and with no risk of adverse effects that accompany pharmacotherapy. With that background, let's learn how to go about forgiving ourselves.

The five steps

Christina, a thirty-two-year-old financial consultant, had significant mental health challenges in her family. The most affected was her younger brother Randy who was in and out of the hospital many times for suicidal ideation. His depression partially responded to the medicines when he took them, which he often didn't. Gradually, he became a recluse. Christina was his only contact with the outside world. She talked to him every evening which helped him get a good night's sleep.

One Saturday, on a date with her boyfriend, Christina put her ringer on vibrate. A few drinks and an evening full of loud music and dance buried Randy's phone call. That night, Randy nearly succeeded in his attempt to take his life.

Christina felt terribly guilty and thought she was selfish. She shouldn't have been at the party when Randy called. Or, at least, she should have set an alarm as a reminder to call him.

Let's apply the five steps of self-forgiveness to Christina's situation. They are modified from a previous self-forgiveness model and inspired by the work of Dr. Luskin.[23]

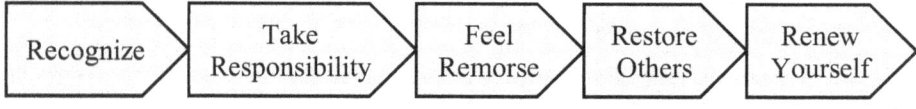

Figure 9. Five steps of self-forgiveness

1. Recognize: In many situations, we rationalize the hurt, sometimes even denying that the other person was injured. Or else, we sometimes create an excuse that they would have been hurt anyway, perhaps even worse, but for our involvement. The first step in self-forgiveness is thus recognizing that the other person was injured and undeservingly so. In Christina's situation, recognition of the hurt (her brother's suicide attempt) was obvious.

2. Take responsibility: You acknowledge that the hurt directly resulted from your words, actions, or inactions. Owning your words, actions, or inactions takes courage and humility, which both make self-forgiveness easier.[24] Christina could try to escape the blame by saying that Randy would have done this anyway, no matter her help. Or she could justify her action by saying that she also deserves to have a life.[25] Both these stances can provide short-term comfort but would not provide long-term healing.

3. Feel remorse: A self-forgiving person genuinely feels bad about what happened. They don't self-forgive because they want to feel lighter. They self-forgive because they care about the person who got hurt.

The path to feeling good goes through feeling bad. You won't feel you deserve your forgiveness unless you feel genuine remorse.

Christina's authentic remorse shows her love for her brother and her desire to do the right thing. It also shows courage and humility in embracing the negative emotions. Remorse often leads to the next step: restoring others.

4. Restore others: You only feel truly worthy if you earned it. The same applies to self-forgiveness. Christina took several actions. She sincerely apologized to her brother and explained to her boyfriend her inability to go on evening dates. She also got another phone exclusively to receive her brother's phone calls, which she would never turn off. Finally, she committed to being more involved in her brother's care so he would improve his compliance with his medicines.

5. Renew yourself: You renew yourself in two ways: instrumentally and emotionally. One, you improve your skillset, so you don't repeat the mistake. Two, you develop humility, courage, and self-compassion, so you are better next time at taking responsibility while maintaining self-worth.[26]

Chaplain Jim Hogg, manager of spiritual care at Trinity Health, an esteemed friend and colleague of mine, very eloquently summarized his years of experience with self-compassion and self-forgiveness in the following words, "Self-forgiveness and self-compassion live near each other. To be able to offer oneself self-compassion includes the ability to offer oneself self-forgiveness. Self-forgiveness is one of the most difficult things to do (and to believe it). Self-compassion flows out of such self-forgiveness. May we ever remember that to forgive oneself is to be compassionate with oneself." I totally echo his words.

As you cultivate greater emotional intelligence, you come to a place of peace with your past. You also develop greater flexibility in thinking. So, while you generally strive to forgive yourself, you recognize that there are situations where self-forgiveness might not work or could actually harm you.

When not to forgive the self

Three situations call for avoiding self-forgiveness.

1. Self-forgiveness may not make sense if you feel guilty or ashamed without doing anything wrong. This often happens to innocent people caught in abusive situations, at work, or in personal life, who feel they somehow are the ones to blame. Parents of children with autism and other medical and psychiatric conditions also often experience uncalled-for guilt and shame.[27] Self-compassion would be more beneficial in this situation.

2. Research shows that situations that call for better behavior control may not be helped by leading with self-forgiveness.[28] For instance, in people trying to quit smoking, try self-compassion instead of self-forgiveness.[29] Similarly, limited research shows that self-forgiveness might predispose to pathological gambling.[30] Having said that, it helps to remember that forces of temptations are hardwired in the human brain. So, you have to be careful balancing self-judgment and self-forgiveness.

3. Premature self-forgiveness for criminal convicts or narcissistic people may also be unhelpful.[31] A person inflicting ongoing harm to the innocent is at risk of continuing their sinister action if they succeed at forgiving themselves prematurely without remorse and building compassion for others. Self-forgiveness is a path to growth and making the other person whole, not putting a lid on one's misdeeds.

I pray you never fall into a situation where you must forgive yourself. I also pray that, if ever needed, self-forgiveness opens a path for you to heal, renew, and grow.

A Covenant With Self

I sincerely hope in the previous pages I was able to convey three truths about our relationship with ourselves:

1. Kindness to oneself is important.
2. We aren't being kind to ourselves.
3. We can develop self-kindness by cultivating greater self-worth and self-love.

Shedding self-rejection, building self-worth, and nurturing self-love offer you a three-step approach to develop a deeper calm, courage, compassion, and connection.

I invite you to pick ideas from each step that resonate with you and find creative ways to bring them to your life. I will continue developing more supportive content (videos, blogs, workbook) that you can access by visiting amitsood.com/tango.

One helpful way you can improve follow-through is by making a covenant. A covenant is a commitment, a binding agreement between two parties with a promise and a responsibility. In signing the covenant, you acknowledge your imperfect past that you are willing to learn from and forgive. Depending on your beliefs, you can consider your covenant sacred (such as the covenants of the Old Testament), or transactional (such as legal covenants).

Please read the items on the next page, and if you feel comfortable, make a commitment and then sign the covenant. Your commitment can be with yourself or with someone else who is close to you.

My heartfelt prayer is for you to forever stay in love with one person who will never leave you lonely — yourself.

YOUR COVENANT

This Covenant dated as of _____ between _____
and _____.

I promise to treat myself with kindness. I promise that despite –

☐ 1. My previous mistakes or failures, I'll stay respectful to myself.

☐ 2. Things not going my way, I'll remain hopeful.

☐ 3. Facing tough times, I'll find reasons for gratitude.

☐ 4. Uncertainty of the results, I'll give my best.

☐ 5. A slow progress, I'll stay patient.

☐ 6. What others think of my looks, I'll feel beautiful inside and outside.

☐ 7. Others' many rejections, I'll continue loving myself.

☐ 8. My several successes, I'll stay humble.

☐ 9. Seeing others doing wrong, I'll do what's right and ethical.

☐ 10. Many fears in my mind, I'll stay courageous.

☐ 11. Seeing others seek short-term success, I'll focus on my long-term purpose.

☐ 12. Many pull to my temptations, I'll stay disciplined and honorable.

☐ 13. Meeting people with different accomplishments, I'll consider everyone equal.

☐ 14. The world mired in war, hatred, and revenge, I'll choose peace, love, and forgiveness.

Signed_____ Signed_____

Epilogue

A few years ago, on a crisp, sunny Minnesotan afternoon, I was privileged to speak to elementary school students in Rochester. The topic was happiness. At the end of the talk, I asked students to name a few things that made them happy. Their responses ranged from ice cream to boogers. One girl raised her hand and spoke words I will never forget. She said, "What makes me happy is that the swing sets work, the grass is soft and green, and the sky is blue." She had come from a land where, because of the smog, she hadn't seen a blue sky until eight years of age.

Her words reminded me of Albert Einstein's thoughts, which I read several years ago. "There are only two ways to live your life. One is as though nothing is a miracle. The other is as though everything is a miracle." Celebrating her wisdom and that of Einstein, I choose the latter, so I can experience the extraordinary within the ordinary.

Friend, you are that extraordinary. Nature has worked extremely hard to endow you with a precious body and a brain that empowers you to talk, think, heal, serve, and love.

I believe you and I aren't a clump of DNA on a random journey to nowhere. Instead, our core, our Esse, is on an intentional ride that entails progressively deepening and widening compassion until no one remains excluded from your love.

The first step to that destination is to develop a healthy and healed relationship with yourself. Healthy self-worth and self-love are essential for nurturing a positive relationship with others, both at home and work. Self-love is also the starting point for a stronger physical body, a creative and productive mind, workplace success, and responsible citizenship.

In this book, through science and stories, I outlined insights and practices to take you one step closer to "Tangoing" with life, alone or with a partner.

I invite you to take the next step now. Convert your learnings and the covenant into a daily practice by starting with a fourteen-day commitment to let your values drive your moments. Each day is focused on one specific practice that takes you closer to shedding self-rejection, building self-worth, and nurturing self-love. Here is one way to do it:

Day 1: Commit to self-respect (despite mistakes or failures)
Day 2: Nurture hope (despite things not going your way)
Day 3: Find reasons for gratitude (despite facing tough times)
Day 4: Give your best (despite the uncertainty of results)
Day 5: Stay patient (despite a slow progress)
Day 6: Feel beautiful (despite what others think of your looks)
Day 7: Love yourself (despite facing rejections)
Day 8: Embrace humility (despite your many successes)
Day 9: Anchor in your core values (despite others doing wrong)
Day 10: Deepen courage (despite your fears)
Day 11: Pursue long-term purpose (despite others seeking short-term gains)
Day 12: Be disciplined and honorable (despite many temptations)
Day 13: Respect everyone (despite people's different achievements)
Day 14: Choose peace, love, and forgiveness (despite living in a world mired in conflicts, hatred, and revenge)

After completing a fourteen-day cycle, you can go back and repeat it or replace a few practices with different ones that work better. Taking a few days' break in between is also totally fine.

Five ways to integrate the practices in your life are reading, thinking, writing, practicing, and sharing.

For example, with day 2 (hope):
1. Read quotes, stories, or books that give you hope.
2. Think about what being hopeful means to you.

3. Write about your experiences and the people in your life who fill you with hope.
4. Look for the positives during the day.
5. Share with a friend or loved one what you learned and practiced.

Working with a like-minded accountability partner to grow together makes the journey even more fun and rewarding. I'm happy to be your partner and toward that end will develop more resources in the coming months and years so we can continue walking together. If you wish, you can visit amitsood.com/tango for more details.

Consider that today is one page in the long trilogy of your life. Write at least one line of humor, kindness, or meaning. You'll enjoy writing the story and reading it on days you may not have much to write.

A few years ago, on a trip to Toronto, I had an amazing conversation with Robbie, my cab driver. I'll forever remember his words which captured the essence of our challenge. Robbie said, "We refuse to accept our divinity." While Robbie came to his conclusions from the angle of faith, his words sum up our current struggles with self-rejection, low self-worth, and the imposter phenomenon.

We are amazing, sacred, pure, and priceless, but in our ignorance and fear, we are unwilling to accept our infinitely precious presence.

Friend, tomorrow, when you wake up and look in the mirror, tell yourself these words:

"I'm an amazing person. I'm proud of myself. I'm unstoppable. The whole world is rooting for me. I choose to keep going. It'll take time and won't be easy. But I'll get there. It'll be marvelous.

If I must cry today to feel better, that's okay. On my toughest days, sometimes, I'll have to cry to find a smile.

No matter how alone I might feel, I'm never lonely. Every person on the planet is my friendly co-traveler. They are all related to me and walking with me. They need me as much as I need them.

I choose to dance so the world can dance with me

Appendix A
Loneliness Basics

Since prehistoric times, loneliness has been our constant companion for a good reason. Loneliness, although unpleasant, is a protective feeling since it motivates us to reach out and connect. Connections are evolutionarily advantageous since they enhance our survival and reproductive success.[1] No wonder the need to belong is integral to the human psyche.[2]

Definition: The feeling of loneliness emerges from unmet connection needs. A popular definition is "a discrepancy between an individual's preferred and actual social relations."[3]

Quality counts: Loneliness has two parts—bad company and no company. Former is worse than the latter.

Loneliness is primarily about individual perception. The same amount and kind of social exposure may be considered caring or exploitative, sufficient or too little, depending on the person.[4]

Further, many of us enjoy being alone. We also enjoy being in a presence where we can be ourselves, feel worthy and respected, have mutual trust, have aligned values and purpose, and mostly do not get bored!

Comedian Robin Williams aptly remarked, "I used to think the worst thing in life was to end up all alone. It's not. The worst thing in life is to end up with people who make you feel all alone." Thus, being alone may not mean feeling lonely, just as being together may not mean feeling connected.

Prevalence: We need no statistics to agree that we are more digitally connected than ever. Yet more than 40 percent of us feel lonely,[5] a feeling that has been steadily increasing since the 1970s based on a review of 345 studies.[6] In some surveys, loneliness prevalence at work has been reported as high as 80 percent.[7]

Causes: Every person's loneliness is unique, and several factors contribute to this feeling in each person. Technological innovations that have led to a change in communication, increased fragmentation of social relationships, and greater mobility opportunities are three reasons compounded by worse mental health. Interestingly, a recent survey showed a direct relationship between the number of meetings and loneliness (the more the number of meetings, the greater the loneliness).[8]

The lingering effect of the pandemic accelerated our loneliness and put many of us in the loneliness trap (detailed in Appendix B).[9] Many of us are lonely because of physical issues (such as hearing or visual impairment), mental disorders, chronic illness, bereavement, retirement, and lack of access to connections (especially seniors, people with disabilities, recent immigrants, those who have been relocated, and people in a new job).[10-11]

Types: Researchers identify three dimensions of connections (and loneliness) — intimate, relational, and collective.[12]

Intimate (or emotional) connections are with one or a few people (spouse, partner, close friend) who support our daily instrumental and emotional needs and are there for us during crises. Lacking such a person or persons creates intimate (or emotional) loneliness.

Friends and family connections comprise our relational dimension (social network; friends or family). They help with "high cost" support such as projects, childcare, and other daily needs. An absence of a high-quality support network causes relational (or social) loneliness.

A collective group includes our workplace, school, sports team, voluntary organization, or other similar larger groups. These groups provide an outer social layer that helps us with our purpose and provides "low-cost" social support. The absence of such a group creates collective loneliness.

Loneliness can also be seen as psychological or contextual, related to a lack of connection or painful disconnection, and a lack of social connections or one's inability to connect.[13]

A final classification is short-term (transient) loneliness that lasts for a few days or weeks, and long-term (chronic) loneliness that lasts for many months or years.

Appendix B
How Loneliness Perpetuates Itself

Short-term loneliness cures itself quickly when we can reach out to caring friends and family. But when we do not have many people we can talk to, then loneliness persists. This persistent loneliness perpetuates itself through two mechanisms: creating a protective reflex and spawning stigma that delays seeking help.

1. Connect or protect?

Loneliness produces two motivations — to connect and to protect.[1-2]

While we mostly badmouth loneliness, I believe loneliness gets an undeserving bad rep. Most of the loneliness-related harms are due to its antecedents, and not because of the unpleasant feeling itself. Loneliness is a protective instinct since a lonely person surrounded by predators is vulnerable. That survival instinct prompts us to find supportive others and stay together — our instinct to connect.

But when loneliness festers for a long time, several changes occur, including in our brains.

We become paranoid about others.[3]

In a social scene, we are more likely to focus on the threatening aspect than someone else not feeling lonely.[4]

We get hypervigilant of others, carry a more negative bias, and look for evidence that confirms our bias.[5]

Lonely individuals' brains process threats at twice the speed of non-lonely persons (116 vs 252 milliseconds).[6]

Lonely individuals do not intentionally try to access the negative information. They can't help it since their focus on social threats is implicit (subconscious).[7] Even in a group, lonely individuals try to maintain a greater distance from others.[8]

The result is that lonely individuals, because of their sensitivity to social threats, start avoiding others.[9-13]

All the above reasons perpetuate loneliness. In this state, even if provided a connection to others, we try to avoid them, a process worsened by the stigma of loneliness.

2. The stigma

A higher proportion of us feel lonely than the number you see in the statistics. This is because, like mental health conditions, loneliness carries a stigma, which is even higher among young people.[14] Further, the higher the loneliness, the greater the stigma, keeping people locked in their shells.[15] Valuing their impression on others, lonely people hide their loneliness to preserve a positive image.[16]

Why the stigma? The reason is simple. Many associate loneliness with being unpopular, weak, poorly adjusted, a low achiever, incompetent, and lacking social skills.[15] This stigma starts in childhood, interfering with developing healthy self-worth since children tend to stigmatize and reject lonely peers.[17] Predictably, stigma decreases the chances of lonely people connecting with others.[18]

Appendix C
Loneliness and Connection with Self

On days we feel really grumpy, many of us want to be left alone. That's a good thing because it takes a superhuman effort to feel kind and connected to others when you are unhappy with yourself. But what would happen if the different types of grumpiness — guilt, shame, self-rejection, low self-worth, lack of self-compassion — stay with you over the long term? In that case, you are likely to be annoyed by people; neither of you will enjoy each other's company.

Below I share a summary of a few research studies that establish the importance of your relationship with yourself in order to have a positive relationship with others.

Guilt and shame
- A study of 505 adolescents and young adults showed that shame was associated with loneliness, and loneliness predisposed to mental health disorders.[1]
- A review of 38 studies involving a more senior population also showed that shame was associated with loneliness.[2]
- In a study of 109 community-dwelling adults with physical limitations, feeling guilty about being a burden was associated with loneliness.[3]
- In another study among 1028 patients with stroke, the more guilty patients felt about being a burden the greater their lonely feelings.[4]

Self-worth
- In a large collaborative review among researchers that looked at ethnic minority and migrant communities, improving self-worth was reported to be among the strongest interventions for improving loneliness.[5]
- In a study among people with substance use disorders, fear of negative evaluation and low self-worth were strongly associated with loneliness.[6]
- In a longitudinal study of 586 children from age 7 to 17 years, low self-worth was associated with persistent loneliness.[7]
- A study of 214 active Facebook users showed that usage with upward comparison was associated with loneliness.[8]
- Another study showed that the use of Instagram for comparison was associated with higher loneliness.[9]

Self-compassion
- Some of the predictors of loneliness aren't modifiable, such as age or gender. Having good people in your life who want to spend time with you is also not always in your hands. However, a study of 2106 people in Belgium showed that high levels of self-compassion (a modifiable factor) were protective against loneliness.[10]
- In a study among older adults, a combination of remotely delivered resilience and self-compassion interventions significantly improved stress, depression, and loneliness.[11]
- Researchers studied 323 adults (mean age of 75 years) to assess the effect of self-compassion on the negative impact of loneliness. Results showed that self-compassion protected people from the adverse effects of loneliness on depression.[12]
- Among 204 Polish citizens, a low rejection sensitivity (a marker of self-compassion), was strongly associated with lower loneliness. Researchers shared the strong link between thoughts and emotions related to oneself and loneliness, with self-compassion serving a protective role. They picked an apt title for the study: "As long as you are self-compassionate, you will never walk alone."[13]
- At a small university in the Southeastern United States, researchers looked at the link between self-compassion and loneliness among 198 undergraduate students. Results showed a moderate negative correlation (self-compassion was protective of loneliness).[14]

- Among U.S. employees, self-compassion was protective of employees experiencing loneliness from feeling depressive symptoms. Researchers aptly called their study, "Depending on your own kindness."[15]
- A study involving 2785 college students showed that self-compassion moderated the association between loneliness and depression.[16]

Self-acceptance
- A study of 415 adults and senior members showed that self-acceptance protected people from the adverse effects of loneliness on well-being.[17]
- People with disabilities of any kind often feel stigmatized, which is a set of unfairly negative beliefs. Many such people carry self-stigma that makes them harsh on themselves because of internalizing negative societal attitudes. In a study involving visually impaired people, self-stigma (which is the opposite of self-acceptance and self-compassion) was significantly associated with loneliness.[18]
- In a study of 257 first-year medical students, 87 percent of students had moderate or high levels of Imposter Phenomenon (IP) at the time of matriculation. IP increased by the time students graduated from their freshman year. High IP was associated with loneliness.[19]

Others
- In a Polish study of 432 participants, emotional intelligence was inversely related to loneliness. Researchers suggested improving emotional intelligence as a fruitful approach to decreasing loneliness.[20]

Appendix D
What Works?

Fortunately, an army of researchers, thinkers, academicians, and others are investigating and implementing approaches that can help mitigate the feeling of loneliness and its downstream consequences.

Unfortunately, the pace of progress in finding and implementing solutions is much slower than the pace of technological innovations pulling us apart.

The technology industry has little regulation and limited guardrails, with an insufficient focus on safety and public good. While healthcare is obsessed with not doing harm and reducing costs to end users, many tech executives think of harm as an afterthought.

With that off my chest, let's summarize several hundred studies evaluating various approaches to improving loneliness. Overall, most approaches show only small to modest benefits, partly because a lifestyle problem that has built over several decades is unlikely to have a quick fix.[1] Below is a summary of the research studies.

Psychological and other social interventions

Providing social skills training, opportunities for social contact, and social support have all been tested and found to have some benefits. None of these approaches are wrong, but they disregard that most people have basic social skills, social contact without removing negative thinking about others is less likely to help, and a bi-directional relationship helps better than receiving uni-directional support for curbing loneliness. Not surprisingly, the most effective solutions have been psychological approaches that help with improving negative thinking.

- A meta-analysis of loneliness-reducing interventions showed that psychoeducation to correct maladaptive cognitions was much more effective than other approaches, such as social skills training or providing social support.[2]
- An analysis of 60 studies showed that counseling-based psychological interventions provided the most benefit.[3]
- An analysis of 31 studies showed that psychological interventions moderately decreased loneliness.[4]
- A review of 15 studies in children and adolescents showed that loneliness was associated with mental health problems longitudinally, and psychological interventions were helpful.[5]
- Approaches that have been somewhat helpful for decreasing loneliness include applying positive past experiences to present relationships, improving coping and stress management techniques, decreasing thought distortion, and removing automatic negative thoughts, false attributions, and self-defeating thoughts.[6-7]
- In a study among older Chinese citizens, psychological interventions had the strongest benefit for reducing loneliness.[8]
- A review of 25 studies among university students showed that social support, social interaction, psychoeducation, and reflective exercises all were helpful. However, the magnitude of the effect was small.[9]

Technology based approaches
- In an analysis of 14 clinical trials, artificial intelligence and large language model-powered relational agents (software programs) decreased loneliness better than studies using social support, social interaction, and social skills improvement programs.[10-11]
- An analysis of 8 clinical trials using social robots showed benefits for reducing loneliness.[12]
- A randomized study among 64 participants using social robots showed benefits for reducing loneliness.[13]
- Technology-based voice assistants are being investigated but haven't provided conclusive positive benefits.[14]
- Several reviews of digital technology interventions, including video call visits, have shown no benefit.[15-17]

- A review of 28 studies showed that communication technologies may reduce loneliness in older adults.[18]
- Another review showed only a modest effect of group-based interventions with a small effect of internet-based strategies among community-dwelling adults.[19]
- Remotely delivered social support and an approach to correct maladaptive social cognition were associated with improved loneliness among older adults.[20]
- Social media connections that enhance real-life connections were helpful for loneliness.[21]
- In users of social networking sites, receiving feedback and likes on one's posts was associated with lower loneliness.[22]

Green space
- A review of 57 studies concluded that the quality of the built environment affects loneliness.[23]
- In a review of 22 studies, researchers examined the association between green spaces and loneliness. Broadly, the study showed that green spaces were protective from loneliness.[24]
- A study of 8049 city dwellers from Australia showed that increasing green spaces to above 10 percent within 1.6 kilometers of home was significantly associated with a reduction in loneliness. This was particularly helpful for people living alone.[25]
- A review of seven studies on place-based interventions suggested the overall effect was generally positive, but more conclusive studies are needed.[26]

Miscellaneous
- A review of 15 studies with seniors showed modest benefits of laughter therapy, horticultural therapy, and reminiscence therapy for decreasing loneliness.[27]
- A review of 70 studies looked at several approaches including pet therapy, psychotherapy or cognitive behavioral therapy, counseling, exercise, music therapy, occupational therapy, reminiscence therapy, social interventions, and technological interventions. Overall, the results showed a small improvement with most approaches. The most powerful effect was with pet therapy.[28]

- A review of 24 studies showed that pet ownership was associated with lower loneliness, with no difference between different types of pets.[29]
- Among 360 teleworkers, dog ownership was associated with more physical activity and lower loneliness.[30]
- A review of 16 studies among patients with cancer showed that mindfulness-based stress reduction (MBSR) was modestly associated with decreased loneliness.[31]

Some of the other approaches that have been modestly beneficial include:
- High-quality listening (decreases the speaker's loneliness).[32]
- Laughter yoga.[33]
- Participation in a chronic disease self-management program.[34]
- Increasing physical touch in relationships.[35]
- Prosocial behavior.[36]
- Home-based interventions among older adults.[37]
- Community programs.[38]
- Helping seniors feel loved.[39]
- Physical exercise.[40]
- Having a sense of purpose in life.[41]

In this section I have not touched the impact of pursuing purpose on loneliness which will merit a much longer discussion. Instead, I would share insight from my friend and colleague, Dr. Heather Farley, Chief Well-being Officer of Medical University at South Carolina, who has been tirelessly advocating for professional well-being, having overcome her own struggles with burnout. In her words, "True joy in work comes not just from what we do, but from the alignment of our work with a deeper sense of purpose. Forming strong connections with colleagues as you work towards a common goal that is larger than oneself is a powerful driver of professional fulfillment."

Notes

Introduction
1. wohasu.com

1. Connect-In
1. Benjamin A. Katz, Jason Karalis, Mariah T. Hawes, Daniel N. Klein, Lonely but not alone: Loneliness and social positive valence sensitivity in emerging adults' everyday lives, Journal of Research in Personality, Volume 109, 2024, 104453.
2. https://blog.perceptyx.com/new-perceptyx-research-shines-a-light-on-loneliness-in-the-workplace (Accessed 07/24/2024)
3. Stavrova, O., & Ren, D. (2023). Alone in a Crowd: Is Social Contact Associated with Less Psychological Pain of Loneliness in Everyday Life?. *Journal of happiness studies, 24*(5), 1841–1860. https://doi.org/10.1007/s10902-023-00661-3
4. Keiner, C., et al. *Acad. Psych.* 2023; Brunes, A., et al. *Health Qual Life Outcomes* 2019
5. Huang, A.R., et al. *J Gerontol A Biol Sci Med Sci* 2024; APA Feb 2024
6. Masi, C. M., Chen, H. Y., Hawkley, L. C., & Cacioppo, J. T. (2011). A meta-analysis of interventions to reduce loneliness. *Personality and social psychology review : an official journal of the Society for Personality and Social Psychology, Inc, 15*(3), 219–266. https://doi.org/10.1177/1088868310377394
7. Thoresen, S., Aakvaag, H. F., Strøm, I. F., Wentzel-Larsen, T., & Birkeland, M. S. (2018). Loneliness as a mediator of the relationship between shame and health problems in young people exposed to childhood violence. *Social science & medicine (1982), 211*, 183–189. https://doi.org/10.1016/j.socscimed.2018.06.002
8. Cohen-Mansfield, J., Hazan, H., Lerman, Y., & Shalom, V. (2016). Correlates and predictors of loneliness in older-adults: a review of quantitative results informed by qualitative insights. *International psychogeriatrics, 28*(4), 557–576. https://doi.org/10.1017/S1041610215001532
9. Pedroso-Chaparro, M. D. S., Cabrera, I., Vara-García, C., Márquez-González, M., & Losada-Baltar, A. (2023). Physical limitations and loneliness: The role of guilt related to self-perception as a burden. *Journal of the American Geriatrics Society, 71*(3), 903–908. https://doi.org/10.1111/jgs.18149
10. Fan, W., Ma, K. K., Yang, C. X., & Guo, Y. L. (2023). The mediating effect of stigma between self-perceived burden and loneliness in stroke patients. *Frontiers in psychiatry, 14*, 1219805. https://doi.org/10.3389/fpsyt.2023.1219805
11. Salway, S., Such, E., Preston, L., Booth, A., Zubair, M., Victor, C., & Raghavan, R. (2020). *Reducing loneliness among migrant and ethnic minority people: a participatory evidence synthesis.* NIHR Journals Library.
12. Ingram, I., Kelly, P. J., Deane, F. P., Baker, A. L., & Dingle, G. A. (2020). Perceptions of loneliness among people accessing treatment for substance use disorders. *Drug and alcohol review, 39*(5), 484–494. https://doi.org/10.1111/dar.13120

13. Qualter, P., Brown, S. L., Rotenberg, K. J., Vanhalst, J., Harris, R. A., Goossens, L., Bangee, M., & Munn, P. (2013). Trajectories of loneliness during childhood and adolescence: predictors and health outcomes. *Journal of adolescence*, *36*(6), 1283–1293. https://doi.org/10.1016/j.adolescence.2013.01.005

14. Dibb, B., & Foster, M. (2021). Loneliness and Facebook use: the role of social comparison and rumination. *Heliyon*, *7*(1), e05999. https://doi.org/10.1016/j.heliyon.2021.e05999

15. Yang C. C. (2016). Instagram Use, Loneliness, and Social Comparison Orientation: Interact and Browse on Social Media, But Don't Compare. *Cyberpsychology, behavior and social networking*, *19*(12), 703–708.https://doi.org/10.1089/cyber.2016.0201

16. Patapoff, M. A., Jester, D. J., Daly, R. E., Mausbach, B. T., Depp, C. A., & Glorioso, D. K. (2024). Remotely-administered resilience and self-compassion intervention targeting loneliness and stress in older adults: a single-case experimental design. *Aging & mental health*, *28*(2), 369–376. https://doi.org/10.1080/13607863.2023.2262411

17. Gao, P., Mosazadeh, H., & Nazari, N. (2023). The Buffering Role of Self-compassion in the Association Between Loneliness with Depressive Symptoms: A Cross-Sectional Survey Study Among Older Adults Living in Residential Care Homes During COVID-19. *International journal of mental health and addiction*, 1–21. Advance online publication. https://doi.org/10.1007/s11469-023-01014-0

18. Borawski, D., & Nowak, A. (2022). As long as you are self-compassionate, you will never walk alone. The interplay between self-compassion and rejection sensitivity in predicting loneliness. *International journal of psychology : Journal international de psychologie*, *57*(5), 621–628. https://doi.org/10.1002/ijop.12850

19. Lyon, Taylor A., "Self-Compassion as a Predictor of Loneliness: The Relationship Between Self-Evaluation Processes and Perceptions of Social Connection" (2015). Selected Honors Theses. Paper 37. https://firescholars.seu.edu/cgi/viewcontent.cgi?article=1038&context=honors

20. Andel, S. A., Shen, W., & Arvan, M. L. (2021). Depending on your own kindness: The moderating role of self-compassion on the within-person consequences of work loneliness during the COVID-19 pandemic. *Journal of occupational health psychology*, *26*(4), 276–290. https://doi.org/10.1037/ocp0000271

21. Wang, S., Tang, Q., Lv, Y., Tao, Y., Liu, X., Zhang, L., & Liu, G. (2023). The Temporal Relationship between Depressive Symptoms and Loneliness: The Moderating Role of Self-Compassion. *Behavioral sciences (Basel, Switzerland)*, *13*(6), 472. https://doi.org/10.3390/bs13060472

22. Wollast, R., Preece, D. A., Schmitz, M., Bigot, A., Gross, J. J., & Luminet, O. (2024). The role of self-compassion in loneliness during the COVID-19 pandemic: a group-based trajectory modelling approach. *Cognition & emotion*, *38*(1), 103–119. https://doi.org/10.1080/02699931.2023.2270201

23. Li, S., Zhang, X., Luo, C., Chen, M., Xie, X., Gong, F., Lv, F., Xu, J., Han, J., Fu, L., & Sun, Y. (2021). The mediating role of self-acceptance in the relationship between loneliness and subjective well-being among the elderly in nursing home: A cross-sectional study. *Medicine*, *100*(40), e27364. https://doi.org/10.1097/MD.0000000000027364

24. Kong, L., Gao, Z., Xu, N., Shao, S., Ma, H., He, Q., Zhang, D., Xu, H., & Qu, H. (2021). The relation between self-stigma and loneliness in visually impaired college students: Self-acceptance as mediator. *Disability and health journal*, *14*(2), 101054. https://doi.org/10.1016/j.dhjo.2020.101054

25. Rosenthal, S., Schlussel, Y., Yaden, M. B., DeSantis, J., Trayes, K., Pohl, C., & Hojat, M. (2021). Persistent Impostor Phenomenon Is Associated With Distress in Medical Students. *Family medicine*, *53*(2), 118–122. https://doi.org/10.22454/FamMed.2021.799997

26. Luo, Q., & Shao, R. (2023). The positive and negative emotion functions related to loneliness: a systematic review of behavioural and neuroimaging studies. *Psychoradiology*, *3*, kkad029. https://doi.org/10.1093/psyrad/kkad029

27. Borawski, D., Sojda, M., Rychlewska, K., & Wajs, T. (2022). Attached but Lonely: Emotional Intelligence as a Mediator and Moderator between Attachment Styles and Loneliness. *International journal of environmental research and public health*, *19*(22), 14831. https://doi.org/10.3390/ijerph192214831

2. RUM
1. Sood, A. (2019). SMART with Dr. Sood. Global Center for Resiliency and Wellbeing.
2. https://www.youtube.com/watch?v=0M-TLhGKgwA&t=13s

3. Your Three Relationships
1. https://www.developmentalscience.com/blog/2017/11/29/teenagers-might-have-a-problem-with-respect-but-its-not-the-one-you-think (Accessed 08/16/2024)
2. Trachtenberg E. (2024). The beneficial effects of social support and prosocial behavior on immunity and health: A psychoneuroimmunology perspective. *Brain, behavior, & immunity - health*, *37*, 100758. https://doi.org/10.1016/j.bbih.2024.100758
3. Holt-Lunstad, J., Smith, T. B., & Layton, J. B. (2010). Social relationships and mortality risk: a meta-analytic review. *PLoS medicine*, *7*(7), e1000316. https://doi.org/10.1371/journal.pmed.1000316
4. Wickramaratne, P. J., Yangchen, T., Lepow, L., Patra, B. G., Glicksburg, B., Talati, A., Adekkanattu, P., Ryu, E., Biernacka, J. M., Charney, A., Mann, J. J., Pathak, J., Olfson, M., & Weissman, M. M.

(2022). Social connectedness as a determinant of mental health: A scoping review. *PLoS one*, *17*(10), e0275004. https://doi.org/10.1371/journal.pone.0275004
5. Office of the Surgeon General (OSG). (2023). *Our Epidemic of Loneliness and Isolation: The U.S. Surgeon General's Advisory on the Healing Effects of Social Connection and Community*. US Department of Health and Human Services.

4. D to C
1. Masi, C. M., Chen, H. Y., Hawkley, L. C., & Cacioppo, J. T. (2011). A meta-analysis of interventions to reduce loneliness. *Personality and social psychology review : an official journal of the Society for Personality and Social Psychology, Inc*, *15*(3), 219–266. https://doi.org/10.1177/1088868310377394
2. Kerr NA, Stanley TB. Revisiting the social stigma of loneliness. *Pers Indiv Differ*. 2021;171:110482.
3. Barreto, M., van Breen, J., Victor, C., Hammond, C., Eccles, A., Richins, M. T., & Qualter, P. (2022). Exploring the nature and variation of the stigma associated with loneliness. *Journal of social and personal relationships*, *39*(9), 2658–2679. https://doi.org/10.1177/02654075221087190
4. https://www.nytimes.com/2021/04/19/well/mind/covid-mental-health-languishing.html (Accessed 7/25/2024)
5. Shields, G. S., Doty, D., Shields, R. H., Gower, G., Slavich, G. M., & Yonelinas, A. P. (2017). Recent life stress exposure is associated with poorer long-term memory, working memory, and self-reported memory. *Stress (Amsterdam, Netherlands)*, *20*(6), 598–607. https://doi.org/10.1080/10253890.2017.1380620
6. Geißler, C. F., Friehs, M. A., Frings, C., & Domes, G. (2023). Time-dependent effects of acute stress on working memory performance: A systematic review and hypothesis. *Psychoneuroendocrinology*, *148*, 105998. https://doi.org/10.1016/j.psyneuen.2022.105998

5. Your Best Friend

6. North Star
1. Hill, P. L., Olaru, G., & Allemand, M. (2023). Do associations between sense of purpose, social support, and loneliness differ across the adult lifespan? *Psychology and Aging, 38*(4), 345–355. https://doi.org/10.1037/pag0000733
2. Macià, D., Cattaneo, G., Solana, J., Tormos, J. M., Pascual-Leone, A., & Bartrés-Faz, D. (2021). Meaning in Life: A Major Predictive Factor for Loneliness Comparable to Health Status and Social Connectedness. *Frontiers in psychology*, *12*, 627547. https://doi.org/10.3389/fpsyg.2021.627547

3. https://en.wikipedia.org/wiki/George_Eastman (Accessed 08/03/2024)

7. Hello Others
1. Andersen, M. L., Araujo, P., Frange, C., & Tufik, S. (2018). Sleep Disturbance and Pain: A Tale of Two Common Problems. *Chest, 154*(5), 1249–1259. https://doi.org/10.1016/j.chest.2018.07.019
2. Boothby, E. J., Cooney, G., Sandstrom, G. M., & Clark, M. S. (2018). The Liking Gap in Conversations: Do People Like Us More Than We Think?. *Psychological science, 29*(11), 1742–1756. https://doi.org/10.1177/0956797618783714
3. Wolf, W., Nafe, A., & Tomasello, M. (2021). The Development of the Liking Gap: Children Older Than 5 Years Think That Partners Evaluate Them Less Positively Than They Evaluate Their Partners. *Psychological science, 32*(5), 789–798. https://doi.org/10.1177/0956797620980754
4. https://www.pewresearch.org/politics/2024/06/24/public-trust-in-government-1958-2024/ (Accessed 7/25/2024)
5. Our Epidemic of Loneliness and Isolation: The U.S. Surgeon General's Advisory on the Healing Effects of Social Connection and Community. 2023

8. Why Self-Rejection?
1. Baumeister, R. F., & Leary, M. R. (1995). The need to belong: desire for interpersonal attachments as a fundamental human motivation. *Psychological bulletin, 117*(3), 497–529.
2. https://www.nber.org/papers/w26345
3. Bravata, D. M., Watts, S. A., Keefer, A. L., Madhusudhan, D. K., Taylor, K. T., Clark, D. M., Nelson, R. S., Cokley, K. O., & Hagg, H. K. (2020). Prevalence, Predictors, and Treatment of Impostor Syndrome: a Systematic Review. *Journal of general internal medicine, 35*(4), 1252–1275. https://doi.org/10.1007/s11606-019-05364-1
4. Ally, B. A., Hussey, E. P., & Donahue, M. J. (2013). A case of hyperthymesia: rethinking the role of the amygdala in autobiographical memory. *Neurocase, 19*(2), 166–181. https://doi.org/10.1080/13554794.2011.654225
5. Colucci-D'Amato, L., Speranza, L., & Volpicelli, F. (2020). Neurotrophic Factor BDNF, Physiological Functions and Therapeutic Potential in Depression, Neurodegeneration and Brain Cancer. *International journal of molecular sciences, 21*(20), 7777. https://doi.org/10.3390/ijms21207777
6. Nilsson, M., Lundh, L. G., & Westling, S. (2022). Childhood maltreatment and self-hatred as distinguishing characteristics of psychiatric patients with self-harm: A comparison with clinical and healthy controls. *Clinical psychology & psychotherapy, 29*(5), 1778–1789. https://doi.org/10.1002/cpp.2744
7. Buecker, S., Mund, M., Chwastek, S., Sostmann, M., & Luhmann, M. (2021). Is loneliness in emerging adults increasing over time? A preregistered cross-temporal meta-analysis and systematic review. *Psychological bulletin, 147*(8), 787–805. https://doi.org/10.1037/bul0000332
8. Surkalim, D. L., Luo, M., Eres, R., Gebel, K., van Buskirk, J., Bauman, A., & Ding, D. (2022). The prevalence of loneliness across 113 countries: systematic review and meta-analysis. *BMJ (Clinical research ed.), 376*, e067068. https://doi.org/10.1136/bmj-2021-067068
9. https://greatergood.berkeley.edu/article/item/four_ways_to_create_high_quality_connections_at_work (accessed August 25th, 2024)
10. https://www.forbes.com/sites/soulaimagourani/2021/05/06/why-most-meetings-fail-before-they-even-begin/?sh=337d8f441096 (Accessed 7/25/2024)
11. https://hbr.org/2017/07/stop-the-meeting-madness (Accessed 7/25/2024)
12. Berscheid, E. (2003). The human's greatest strength: Other humans. In L. G Aspinwall, & U. M. Staudinger (Eds.), A psychology of human strengths (pp. 37-48). Washington, DC: American Psychological Association.
13. https://www.usatoday.com/money/blueprint/pet-insurance/animal-abuse-statistics/#sources (Accessed 7/25/2024)

14. https://www.npr.org/sections/goatsandsoda/2022/09/13/1122714064/modern-slavery-global-estimate-increase (Accessed 7/25/2024)
15. Flynn, F. J., & Schaumberg, R. L. (2012). When feeling bad leads to feeling good: guilt-proneness and affective organizational commitment. *The Journal of applied psychology*, *97*(1), 124–133. https://doi.org/10.1037/a0024166

9. Guilt (and Shame)

1. Szentágotai-Tătar, A., & Miu, A. C. (2016). Individual Differences in Emotion Regulation, Childhood Trauma and Proneness to Shame and Guilt in Adolescence. *PloS one*, *11*(11), e0167299. https://doi.org/10.1371/journal.pone.0167299
2. Cândea, D. M., & Szentagotai-Tătar, A. (2018). Shame-proneness, guilt-proneness and anxiety symptoms: A meta-analysis. *Journal of anxiety disorders*, *58*, 78–106. https://doi.org/10.1016/j.janxdis.2018.07.005
3. Shen L. (2018). The evolution of shame and guilt. *PloS one*, *13*(7), e0199448. https://doi.org/10.1371/journal.pone.0199448
4. Giorgetta, C., Strappini, F., Capuozzo, A., Evangelista, E., Magno, A., Castelfranchi, C., & Mancini, F. (2023). Guilt, shame, and embarrassment: similar or different emotions? A comparison between Italians and Americans. *Frontiers in psychology*, *14*, 1260396. https://doi.org/10.3389/fpsyg.2023.1260396
5. Patock-Peckham, J. A., Canning, J. R., & Leeman, R. F. (2018). Shame is bad and guilt is good: An examination of the impaired control over drinking pathway to alcohol use and related problems. *Personality and individual differences*, *121*, 62–66. https://doi.org/10.1016/j.paid.2017.09.023
6. Dickerson, S. S., Kemeny, M. E., Aziz, N., Kim, K. H., & Fahey, J. L. (2004). Immunological effects of induced shame and guilt. *Psychosomatic medicine*, *66*(1), 124–131. https://doi.org/10.1097/01.psy.0000097338.75454.29
7. Szentágotai-Tătar, A., & Miu, A. C. (2016). Individual Differences in Emotion Regulation, Childhood Trauma and Proneness to Shame and Guilt in Adolescence. *PloS one*, *11*(11), e0167299. https://doi.org/10.1371/journal.pone.0167299
8. Fergus, T. A., Valentiner, D. P., McGrath, P. B., & Jencius, S. (2010). Shame- and guilt-proneness: relationships with anxiety disorder symptoms in a clinical sample. *Journal of anxiety disorders*, *24*(8), 811–815. https://doi.org/10.1016/j.janxdis.2010.06.002
9. VanDerhei, S., Rojahn, J., Stuewig, J., & McKnight, P. E. (2014). The effect of shame-proneness, guilt-proneness, and internalizing tendencies on nonsuicidal self-injury. *Suicide & life-threatening behavior*, *44*(3), 317–330. https://doi.org/10.1111/sltb.12069
10. https://journals.sagepub.com/doi/abs/10.1177/0146167211435796
11. Martinez, A. G., Stuewig, J., & Tangney, J. P. (2014). Can perspective-taking reduce crime? Examining a pathway through empathic-concern and guilt-proneness. *Personality & social psychology bulletin*, *40*(12), 1659–1667. https://doi.org/10.1177/0146167214554915
12. Szentágotai-Tătar, A., Chiş, A., Vulturar, R., Dobrean, A., Cândea, D. M., & Miu, A. C. (2015). Shame and Guilt-Proneness in Adolescents: Gene-Environment Interactions. *PloS one*, *10*(7), e0134716. https://doi.org/10.1371/journal.pone.0134716
13. Craven, M. P., & Fekete, E. M. (2019). Weight-related shame and guilt, intuitive eating, and binge eating in female college students. *Eating behaviors*, *33*, 44–48. https://doi.org/10.1016/j.eatbeh.2019.03.002
14. Cavalera, C., Pepe, A., Zurloni, V., Diana, B., Realdon, O., Todisco, P., Castelnuovo, G., Molinari, E., & Pagnini, F. (2018). Negative social emotions and cognition: Shame, guilt and working memory impairments. *Acta psychologica*, *188*, 9–15. https://doi.org/10.1016/j.actpsy.2018.05.005
15. Bub, K., & Lommen, M. J. J. (2017). The role of guilt in Posttraumatic Stress Disorder. *European journal of psychotraumatology*, *8*(1), 1407202. https://doi.org/10.1080/20008198.2017.1407202
16. Leach, C. W., & Cidam, A. (2015). When is shame linked to constructive approach orientation? A meta-analysis. *Journal of personality and social psychology*, *109*(6), 983–1002. https://doi.org/10.1037/pspa0000037

17. Ypsilanti, A., Gettings, R., Lazaras, L., Robson, A., Powell, P. A., & Overton, P. G. (2020). Self-Disgust Is Associated With Loneliness, Mental Health Difficulties, and Eye-Gaze Avoidance in War Veterans With PTSD. *Frontiers in psychology*, *11*, 559883. https://doi.org/10.3389/fpsyg.2020.559883
18. Ypsilanti, A., Robson, A., Lazuras, L., Powell, P. A., & Overton, P. G. (2020). Self-disgust, loneliness and mental health outcomes in older adults: An eye-tracking study. *Journal of affective disorders*, *266*, 646–654. https://doi.org/10.1016/j.jad.2020.01.166
19. Clarke, A., Simpson, J., & Varese, F. (2019). A systematic review of the clinical utility of the concept of self-disgust. *Clinical psychology & psychotherapy*, *26*(1), 110–134. https://doi.org/10.1002/cpp.2335
20. Hirao, K., & Kobayashi, R. (2013). The relationship between self-disgust, guilt, and flow experience among Japanese undergraduates. *Neuropsychiatric disease and treatment*, *9*, 985–988. https://doi.org/10.2147/NDT.S46895
21. Mason, D., James, D., Andrew, L., & Fox, J. R. E. (2022). 'The last thing you feel is the self-disgust'. The role of self-directed disgust in men who have attempted suicide: A grounded theory study. *Psychology and psychotherapy*, *95*(2), 575–599. https://doi.org/10.1111/papt.12389
22. Brake, C. A., Rojas, S. M., Badour, C. L., Dutton, C. E., & Feldner, M. T. (2017). Self-disgust as a potential mechanism underlying the association between PTSD and suicide risk. *Journal of anxiety disorders*, *47*, 1–9. https://doi.org/10.1016/j.janxdis.2017.01.003
23. Ille, R., Schöggl, H., Kapfhammer, H. P., Arendasy, M., Sommer, M., & Schienle, A. (2014). Self-disgust in mental disorders -- symptom-related or disorder-specific?. *Comprehensive psychiatry*, *55*(4), 938–943. https://doi.org/10.1016/j.comppsych.2013.12.020
24. Gao, S., Zhang, L., Yao, X., Lin, J., & Meng, X. (2022). Associations between self-disgust, depression, and anxiety: A three-level meta-analytic review. *Acta psychologica*, *228*, 103658. https://doi.org/10.1016/j.actpsy.2022.103658

10. Taming Your Guilt (and Shame)
1. van Dijk, W. W., van Dillen, L. F., Rotteveel, M., & Seip, E. C. (2017). Looking into the crystal ball of our emotional lives: emotion regulation and the overestimation of future guilt and shame. *Cognition & emotion*, *31*(3), 616–624. https://doi.org/10.1080/02699931.2015.1129313
2. Fougnie, D., & Marois, R. (2006). Distinct capacity limits for attention and working memory: Evidence from attentive tracking and visual working memory paradigms. *Psychological science*, *17*(6), 526–534. https://doi.org/10.1111/j.1467-9280.2006.01739.x
3. Marois, R., & Ivanoff, J. (2005). Capacity limits of information processing in the brain. *Trends in cognitive sciences*, *9*(6), 296–305. https://doi.org/10.1016/j.tics.2005.04.010
4. Reimer, C. B., & Schubert, T. (2020). Visual and central attention share a capacity limitation when the demands for serial item selection in visual search are high. *Attention, perception & psychophysics*, *82*(2), 715–728. https://doi.org/10.3758/s13414-019-01903-4

11. Knowing Self-worth
1. Orth, U., Maes, J., & Schmitt, M. (2015). Self-esteem development across the life span: a longitudinal study with a large sample from Germany. *Developmental psychology*, *51*(2), 248–259. https://doi.org/10.1037/a0038481
2. Orth, U., Trzesniewski, K. H., & Robins, R. W. (2010). Self-esteem development from young adulthood to old age: a cohort-sequential longitudinal study. *Journal of personality and social psychology*, *98*(4), 645–658. https://doi.org/10.1037/a0018769
3. Crocker, J., & Park, L. E. (2004). The costly pursuit of self-esteem. *Psychological bulletin*, *130*(3), 392–414. https://doi.org/10.1037/0033-2909.130.3.392
4. Park, L. E., Ward, D. E., & Naragon-Gainey, K. (2017). It's All About the Money (For Some): Consequences of Financially Contingent Self-Worth. *Personality & social psychology bulletin*, *43*(5), 601–622. https://doi.org/10.1177/0146167216689080
5. Crocker, J., Karpinski, A., Quinn, D. M., & Chase, S. K. (2003). When grades determine self-worth: consequences of contingent self-worth for male and female engineering and psychology majors.

Journal of personality and social psychology, *85*(3), 507–516. https://doi.org/10.1037/0022-3514.85.3.507
6. Luhtanen, R. K., & Crocker, J. (2005). Alcohol use in college students: effects of level of self-esteem, narcissism, and contingencies of self-worth. *Psychology of addictive behaviors : journal of the Society of Psychologists in Addictive Behaviors*, *19*(1), 99–103. https://doi.org/10.1037/0893-164X.19.1.99
7. Ishizu K. (2017). Contingent self-worth moderates the relationship between school stressors and psychological stress responses. *Journal of adolescence*, *56*, 113–117. https://doi.org/10.1016/j.adolescence.2017.02.008

12. Why did I Forget?
1. Covington, M. V., & Beery, R. G. (1976). *Self-worth and school learning.* Oxford, U K: Holt, Rinehart & Winston.

13. Our Comparison Instinct
1. Festinger, L. (1954). A theory of social comparison processes. *Human Relations, 7*, 117–140.
2. Loyalka, P., Zakharov, A., & Kuzima, Y. Catching the Big Fish in the Little Pond Effect: Evidence from 33 Countries and Regions. *Comparative Education Review*, 2018 62:4, 542-564
3. Dumas, F., Fagot, J., Davranche, K., & Claidière, N. (2017). Other better versus self better in baboons: an evolutionary approach of social comparison. *Proceedings. Biological sciences*, *284*(1855), 20170248. https://doi.org/10.1098/rspb.2017.0248
4. Brosnan, S. F., & De Waal, F. B. (2003). Monkeys reject unequal pay. *Nature*, *425*(6955), 297–299. https://doi.org/10.1038/nature01963
5. Manger, T., & Eikeland, O. J. (1997). The effect of social comparison on mathematics self-concept. *Scandinavian journal of psychology*, *38*(3), 237–241. https://doi.org/10.1111/1467-9450.00032
6. Villanueva-Moya, L., Herrera, M. C., Sánchez-Hernández, M. D., & Expósito, F. (2023). #Instacomparison: Social Comparison and Envy as Correlates of Exposure to Instagram and Cyberbullying Perpetration. *Psychological reports*, *126*(3), 1284–1304. https://doi.org/10.1177/00332941211067390
7. Prieler, M., Choi, J., & Lee, H. E. (2021). The Relationships among Self-Worth Contingency on Others' Approval, Appearance Comparisons on Facebook, and Adolescent Girls' Body Esteem: A Cross-Cultural Study. *International journal of environmental research and public health*, *18*(3), 901. https://doi.org/10.3390/ijerph18030901
8. Pedalino, F., & Camerini, A. L. (2022). Instagram Use and Body Dissatisfaction: The Mediating Role of Upward Social Comparison with Peers and Influencers among Young Females. *International journal of environmental research and public health*, *19*(3), 1543. https://doi.org/10.3390/ijerph19031543

14. Hurtful Comparisons
1. Sánchez-Hernández, M. D., Herrera, M. C., & Expósito, F. (2022). Does the Number of Likes Affect Adolescents' Emotions? The Moderating Role of Social Comparison and Feedback-Seeking on Instagram. *The Journal of psychology*, *156*(3), 200–223. https://doi.org/10.1080/00223980.2021.2024120
2. Jung, W. H., & Kim, H. (2020). Intrinsic Functional and Structural Brain Connectivity in Humans Predicts Individual Social Comparison Orientation. *Frontiers in psychiatry*, *11*, 809. https://doi.org/10.3389/fpsyt.2020.00809
3. Fassl, F., Yanagida, T., & Kollmayer, M. (2020). Impostors Dare to Compare: Associations Between the Impostor Phenomenon, Gender Typing, and Social Comparison Orientation in University Students. *Frontiers in psychology*, *11*, 1225. https://doi.org/10.3389/fpsyg.2020.01225
4. Okano, H., & Nomura, M. (2023). Examining social anxiety and dual aspects of social comparison orientation: the moderating role of self-evaluation of social skills. *Frontiers in psychology*, *14*, 1270143. https://doi.org/10.3389/fpsyg.2023.1270143

5. Stefana, A., Dakanalis, A., Mura, M., Colmegna, F., & Clerici, M. (2022). Instagram Use and Mental Well-Being: The Mediating Role of Social Comparison. *The Journal of nervous and mental disease*, *210*(12), 960–965. https://doi.org/10.1097/NMD.0000000000001577

6. Weiguo, Z., Wen, D., Qingtian, L., Xinning, W., & Ming, Z. (2022). Compared with Him or Her, I Am Not Good Enough: How to Alleviate Depression Due to Upward Social Comparison?. *The Journal of psychology*, *156*(7), 512–534. https://doi.org/10.1080/00223980.2022.2101421

7. Stefana, A., Dakanalis, A., Mura, M., Colmegna, F., & Clerici, M. (2022). Instagram Use and Mental Well-Being: The Mediating Role of Social Comparison. *The Journal of nervous and mental disease*, *210*(12), 960–965. https://doi.org/10.1097/NMD.0000000000001577

8. Hu, Y. T., Liu, Q. Q., & Ma, Z. F. (2023). Does Upward Social Comparison on SNS Inspire Adolescent Materialism? Focusing on the Role of Self-Esteem and Mindfulness. *The Journal of psychology*, *157*(1), 32–47. https://doi.org/10.1080/00223980.2022.2134277

9. Kim, H., Schlicht, R., Schardt, M., & Florack, A. (2021). The contributions of social comparison to social network site addiction. *PloS one*, *16*(10), e0257795. https://doi.org/10.1371/journal.pone.0257795

10. Hawes, T., Zimmer-Gembeck, M. J., & Campbell, S. M. (2020). Unique associations of social media use and online appearance preoccupation with depression, anxiety, and appearance rejection sensitivity. *Body image*, *33*, 66–76. https://doi.org/10.1016/j.bodyim.2020.02.010

11. Jarman, H. K., Marques, M. D., McLean, S. A., Slater, A., & Paxton, S. J. (2021). Social media, body satisfaction and well-being among adolescents: A mediation model of appearance-ideal internalization and comparison. *Body image*, *36*, 139–148. https://doi.org/10.1016/j.bodyim.2020.11.005

12. McCarthy, P. A., & Morina, N. (2020). Exploring the association of social comparison with depression and anxiety: A systematic review and meta-analysis. *Clinical psychology & psychotherapy*, *27*(5), 640–671. https://doi.org/10.1002/cpp.2452

13. Nesi, J., & Prinstein, M. J. (2015). Using Social Media for Social Comparison and Feedback-Seeking: Gender and Popularity Moderate Associations with Depressive Symptoms. *Journal of abnormal child psychology*, *43*(8), 1427–1438. https://doi.org/10.1007/s10802-015-0020-0

15. Helpful Comparisons

1. Gable, S. L., Reis, H. T., Impett, E. A., & Asher, E. R. (2004). What do you do when things go right? The intrapersonal and interpersonal benefits of sharing positive events. *Journal of personality and social psychology*, *87*(2), 228–245. https://doi.org/10.1037/0022-3514.87.2.228

2. Gosnell, C. L., & Gable, S. L. (2013). Attachment and capitalizing on positive events. *Attachment & human development*, *15*(3), 281–302. https://doi.org/10.1080/14616734.2013.782655

3. Gable, S. L., Gonzaga, G. C., & Strachman, A. (2006). Will you be there for me when things go right? Supportive responses to positive event disclosures. *Journal of personality and social psychology*, *91*(5), 904–917. https://doi.org/10.1037/0022-3514.91.5.904

4. Yang, C. C., Holden, S. M., Carter, M. D. K., & Webb, J. J. (2018). Social media social comparison and identity distress at the college transition: A dual-path model. *Journal of adolescence*, *69*, 92–102. https://doi.org/10.1016/j.adolescence.2018.09.007

5. Pavlova, M. K., Lechner, C. M., & Silbereisen, R. K. (2018). Social Comparison in Coping With Occupational Uncertainty: Self-Improvement, Self-Enhancement, and the Regional Context. *Journal of personality*, *86*(2), 320–333. https://doi.org/10.1111/jopy.12317

6. Kampmann, I. L., Meyer, T., & Morina, N. (2020). Social comparison modulates coping with fear in virtual environments. *Journal of anxiety disorders*, *72*, 102226. https://doi.org/10.1016/j.janxdis.2020.102226

7. Rheu, M., Peng, W., & Haung, K. T. (2023). Leveraging Upward Social Comparison in Social Media to Promote Healthy Parenting. *Health communication*, *38*(2), 205–215. https://doi.org/10.1080/10410236.2021.1943891

8. Zhang, J., Brackbill, D., Yang, S., Becker, J., Herbert, N., & Centola, D. (2016). Support or competition? How online social networks increase physical activity: A randomized controlled trial. *Preventive medicine reports*, *4*, 453–458. https://doi.org/10.1016/j.pmedr.2016.08.008

9. Rheu, M., Peng, W., & Haung, K. T. (2023). Leveraging Upward Social Comparison in Social Media to Promote Healthy Parenting. *Health communication*, *38*(2), 205–215. https://doi.org/10.1080/10410236.2021.1943891

10. van Harreveld, F., van der Pligt, J., & Nordgren, L. (2008). The relativity of bad decisions: social comparison as a means to alleviate regret. *The British journal of social psychology*, *47*(Pt 1), 105–117. https://doi.org/10.1348/014466607X260134

11. Orth, U., Maes, J., & Schmitt, M. (2015). Self-esteem development across the life span: a longitudinal study with a large sample from Germany. *Developmental psychology*, *51*(2), 248–259. https://doi.org/10.1037/a0038481

12. Robins, R. W., Trzesniewski, K. H., Tracy, J. L., Gosling, S. D., & Potter, J. (2002). Global self-esteem across the life span. *Psychology and aging*, *17*(3), 423–434.

13. Orth, U., Robins, R. W., & Widaman, K. F. (2012). Life-span development of self-esteem and its effects on important life outcomes. *Journal of personality and social psychology*, *102*(6), 1271–1288. https://doi.org/10.1037/a0025558

14. Orth, U., Trzesniewski, K. H., & Robins, R. W. (2010). Self-esteem development from young adulthood to old age: a cohort-sequential longitudinal study. *Journal of personality and social psychology*, *98*(4), 645–658. https://doi.org/10.1037/a0018769

15. Solmi, M., Radua, J., Olivola, M., Croce, E., Soardo, L., Salazar de Pablo, G., Il Shin, J., Kirkbride, J. B., Jones, P., Kim, J. H., Kim, J. Y., Carvalho, A. F., Seeman, M. V., Correll, C. U., & Fusar-Poli, P. (2022). Age at onset of mental disorders worldwide: large-scale meta-analysis of 192 epidemiological studies. *Molecular psychiatry*, *27*(1), 281–295. https://doi.org/10.1038/s41380-021-01161-7

16. Understanding Self-love

1. Garmany, A., Yamada, S., & Terzic, A. (2021). Longevity leap: mind the healthspan gap. *NPJ Regenerative medicine*, *6*(1), 57. https://doi.org/10.1038/s41536-021-00169-5

2. Milman, S., & Barzilai, N. (2023). Discovering Biological Mechanisms of Exceptional Human Health Span and Life Span. *Cold Spring Harbor perspectives in medicine*, *13*(9), a041204. https://doi.org/10.1101/cshperspect.a041204

3. Sheldon, K. M., Corcoran, M., & Sheldon, M. (2021). Duchenne Smiles as Honest Signals of Chronic Positive Mood. *Perspectives on psychological science : a journal of the Association for Psychological Science*, *16*(3), 654–666. https://doi.org/10.1177/1745691620959831

4. Gunnery, S. D., & Ruben, M. A. (2016). Perceptions of Duchenne and non-Duchenne smiles: A meta-analysis. *Cognition & emotion*, *30*(3), 501–515. https://doi.org/10.1080/02699931.2015.1018817

17. Say No to Life Limiters

1. Magnan S. Social determinants of health 101 for health care: five plus five. *NAM Perspectives*. Washington, DC: National Academy of Medicine; 2017.

2. https://nam.edu/social-determinants-of-health-101-for-health-care-five-plus-five. Accessed 7/25/2024

3. Gao, W., Sanna, M., Chen, Y. H., Tsai, M. K., & Wen, C. P. (2024). Occupational Sitting Time, Leisure Physical Activity, and All-Cause and Cardiovascular Disease Mortality. *JAMA network open*, *7*(1), e2350680. https://doi.org/10.1001/jamanetworkopen.2023.50680

4. Bailey, D. P., Hewson, D. J., Champion, R. B., & Sayegh, S. M. (2019). Sitting Time and Risk of Cardiovascular Disease and Diabetes: A Systematic Review and Meta-Analysis. *American journal of preventive medicine*, *57*(3), 408–416. https://doi.org/10.1016/j.amepre.2019.04.015

5. Levine J. A. (2015). Sick of sitting. *Diabetologia*, *58*(8), 1751–1758. https://doi.org/10.1007/s00125-015-3624-6

6. Hermelink, R., Leitzmann, M. F., Markozannes, G., Tsilidis, K., Pukrop, T., Berger, F., Baurecht, H., & Jochem, C. (2022). Sedentary behavior and cancer-an umbrella review and meta-analysis. *European journal of epidemiology*, *37*(5), 447–460. https://doi.org/10.1007/s10654-022-00873-6

7. Basu, N., Yang, X., Luben, R. N., Whibley, D., Macfarlane, G. J., Wareham, N. J., Khaw, K. T., & Myint, P. K. (2016). Fatigue is associated with excess mortality in the general population: results from the EPIC-Norfolk study. *BMC medicine*, *14*(1), 122. https://doi.org/10.1186/s12916-016-0662-y

8. Chapman, B. P., Fiscella, K., Kawachi, I., Duberstein, P., & Muennig, P. (2013). Emotion suppression and mortality risk over a 12-year follow-up. *Journal of psychosomatic research*, *75*(4), 381–385. https://doi.org/10.1016/j.jpsychores.2013.07.014

9. Mostofsky, E., Maclure, M., Tofler, G. H., Muller, J. E., & Mittleman, M. A. (2013). Relation of outbursts of anger and risk of acute myocardial infarction. *The American journal of cardiology*, *112*(3), 343–348. https://doi.org/10.1016/j.amjcard.2013.03.035

10. Kim, E. S., Hagan, K. A., Grodstein, F., DeMeo, D. L., De Vivo, I., & Kubzansky, L. D. (2017). Optimism and Cause-Specific Mortality: A Prospective Cohort Study. *American journal of epidemiology*, *185*(1), 21–29. https://doi.org/10.1093/aje/kww182

11. Rico-Uribe, L. A., Caballero, F. F., Martín-María, N., Cabello, M., Ayuso-Mateos, J. L., & Miret, M. (2018). Association of loneliness with all-cause mortality: A meta-analysis. *PloS one*, *13*(1), e0190033. https://doi.org/10.1371/journal.pone.0190033

12. Baumeister, R. F., & Leary, M. R. (1995). The need to belong: desire for interpersonal attachments as a fundamental human motivation. *Psychological bulletin*, *117*(3), 497–529.

13. Collins, H. K., Hagerty, S. F., Quoidbach, J., Norton, M. I., & Brooks, A. W. (2022). Relational diversity in social portfolios predicts well-being. *Proceedings of the National Academy of Sciences of the United States of America*, *119*(43), e2120668119. https://doi.org/10.1073/pnas.2120668119

14. Hill, P. L., Olaru, G., & Allemand, M. (2023). Do associations between sense of purpose, social support, and loneliness differ across the adult lifespan? *Psychology and Aging*, *38*(4), 345–355. https://doi.org/10.1037/pag0000733

18. Self, an Introduction

1. Brewer, J. A., Garrison, K. A., & Whitfield-Gabrieli, S. (2013). What about the "Self" is Processed in the Posterior Cingulate Cortex?. *Frontiers in human neuroscience*, *7*, 647. https://doi.org/10.3389/fnhum.2013.00647

2. Garrison, K. A., Santoyo, J. F., Davis, J. H., Thornhill, T. A., 4th, Kerr, C. E., & Brewer, J. A. (2013). Effortless awareness: using real time neurofeedback to investigate correlates of posterior cingulate cortex activity in meditators' self-report. *Frontiers in human neuroscience*, *7*, 440. https://doi.org/10.3389/fnhum.2013.00440

3. Palhano-Fontes, F., Andrade, K. C., Tofoli, L. F., Santos, A. C., Crippa, J. A., Hallak, J. E., Ribeiro, S., & de Araujo, D. B. (2015). The psychedelic state induced by ayahuasca modulates the activity and connectivity of the default mode network. *PloS one*, *10*(2), e0118143. https://doi.org/10.1371/journal.pone.0118143

4. Carhart-Harris, R. L., Erritzoe, D., Williams, T., Stone, J. M., Reed, L. J., Colasanti, A., Tyacke, R. J., Leech, R., Malizia, A. L., Murphy, K., Hobden, P., Evans, J., Feilding, A., Wise, R. G., & Nutt, D. J. (2012). Neural correlates of the psychedelic state as determined by fMRI studies with psilocybin. *Proceedings of the National Academy of Sciences of the United States of America*, *109*(6), 2138–2143. https://doi.org/10.1073/pnas.1119598109

5. Levorsen, M., Aoki, R., Matsumoto, K., Sedikides, C., & Izuma, K. (2023). The Self-Concept Is Represented in the Medial Prefrontal Cortex in Terms of Self-Importance. *The Journal of neuroscience : the official journal of the Society for Neuroscience*, *43*(20), 3675–3686. https://doi.org/10.1523/JNEUROSCI.2178-22.2023

6. Haruki, Y., & Ogawa, K. (2021). Role of anatomical insular subdivisions in interoception: Interoceptive attention and accuracy have dissociable substrates. *The European journal of neuroscience*, *53*(8), 2669–2680. https://doi.org/10.1111/ejn.15157

7. Brown N. R. (2023). Autobiographical memory and the self: A transition theory perspective. *Wiley interdisciplinary reviews. Cognitive science*, *14*(3), e1621. https://doi.org/10.1002/wcs.1621
8. Binder, J. R., & Desai, R. H. (2011). The neurobiology of semantic memory. *Trends in cognitive sciences*, *15*(11), 527–536. https://doi.org/10.1016/j.tics.2011.10.001
9. Interview with Michael Gazzaniga. (2011). *Annals of the New York Academy of Sciences*, *1224*, 1–8. https://doi.org/10.1111/j.1749-6632.2011.05998.x
10. Baumeister, R. F. (2022). The Self Explained. Why and How We Become Who We Are. Guilford Publications.

19. Build or break?

20. What Do You Think?
1. https://www.theatlantic.com/science/archive/2019/07/underappreciated-power-apollo-computer/594121/ Accessed 7/25/2024
2. https://www.npr.org/templates/story/story.php?storyId=124007551#:~:text=Most%20Americans%20Do%20A%20survey,the%20widespread%20belief%20in%20miracles. Accessed 7/25/2024

21. Your Presence
1. Willis, J., & Todorov, A. (2006). First impressions: making up your mind after a 100-ms exposure to a face. *Psychological science*, *17*(7), 592–598. https://doi.org/10.1111/j.1467-9280.2006.01750.x
2. Pandeirada, J. N. S., Fernandes, N. L., Madeira, M., Marinho, P. I., & Vasconcelos, M. (2022). Can I Trust This Person? Evaluations of Trustworthiness From Faces and Relevant Individual Variables. *Frontiers in psychology*, *13*, 857511. https://doi.org/10.3389/fpsyg.2022.857511

22. Our Complex Psyche
1. https://www.nytimes.com/2019/05/28/smarter-living/you-accomplished-something-great-so-now-what.html Accessed 7/25/2024
2. Gilbert, D. T., Pinel, E. C., Wilson, T. D., Blumberg, S. J., & Wheatley, T. P. (1998). Immune neglect: A source of durability bias in affective forecasting. *Journal of Personality and Social Psychology*, *75*(3), 617–638.
3. Madigan, S., Deneault, A. A., Racine, N., Park, J., Thiemann, R., Zhu, J., Dimitropoulos, G., Williamson, T., Fearon, P., Cénat, J. M., McDonald, S., Devereux, C., & Neville, R. D. (2023). Adverse childhood experiences: a meta-analysis of prevalence and moderators among half a million adults in 206 studies. *World psychiatry : official journal of the World Psychiatric Association (WPA)*, *22*(3), 463–471. https://doi.org/10.1002/wps.21122

23. What is Self-Compassion?
1. Singer, T., & Klimecki, O. M. (2014). Empathy and compassion. *Current biology : CB*, *24*(18), R875–R878. https://doi.org/10.1016/j.cub.2014.06.054
2. Klimecki, O. M., Leiberg, S., Ricard, M., & Singer, T. (2014). Differential pattern of functional brain plasticity after compassion and empathy training. *Social cognitive and affective neuroscience*, *9*(6), 873–879. https://doi.org/10.1093/scan/nst060
3. Topçu, N., Akbolat, M., & Amarat, M. (2023). The mediating role of empathy in the impact of compassion fatigue on burnout among nurses. *Journal of research in nursing : JRN*, *28*(6-7), 485–495. *Canadian veterinary journal = La revue veterinaire canadienne*, *59*(7), 749–750. https://doi.org/10.1177/17449871231177164; Dowling T. (2018). Compassion does not fatigue!. *The*
4. Strauss, C., Lever Taylor, B., Gu, J., Kuyken, W., Baer, R., Jones, F., & Cavanagh, K. (2016). What is compassion and how can we measure it? A review of definitions and measures. *Clinical psychology review*, *47*, 15–27. https://doi.org/10.1016/j.cpr.2016.05.004

5. Goldin, P. R., McRae, K., Ramel, W., & Gross, J. J. (2008). The neural bases of emotion regulation: reappraisal and suppression of negative emotion. *Biological psychiatry*, *63*(6), 577–586. https://doi.org/10.1016/j.biopsych.2007.05.031

6. Marcks, B. A., & Woods, D. W. (2005). A comparison of thought suppression to an acceptance-based technique in the management of personal intrusive thoughts: a controlled evaluation. *Behaviour research and therapy*, *43*(4), 433–445. https://doi.org/10.1016/j.brat.2004.03.005

7. Ryckman, N. A., Addis, D. R., Latham, A. J., & Lambert, A. J. (2018). Forget about the future: effects of thought suppression on memory for imaginary emotional episodes. *Cognition & emotion*, *32*(1), 200–206. https://doi.org/10.1080/02699931.2016.1276049

8. Symonides, B., Holas, P., Schram, M., Śleszycka, J., Bogaczewicz, A., & Gaciong, Z. (2014). Does the control of negative emotions influence blood pressure control and its variability?. *Blood pressure*, *23*(6), 323–329. https://doi.org/10.3109/08037051.2014.901006

9. Glück J. (2024). Wisdom and aging. *Current opinion in psychology*, *55*, 101742. https://doi.org/10.1016/j.copsyc.2023.101742

10. https://wisdomcenter.uchicago.edu/news/wisdom-news/are-older-people-wiser Accessed 7/25/2024

24. Common Barriers to Self-Compassion

1. Robinson, K. J., Mayer, S., Allen, A. B., Terry, M., Chilton, A., & Leary, M. R. (2016). Resisting self-compassion: Why are some people opposed to being kind to themselves? *Self and Identity*, *15*(5), 505–524.

2. Zhang, H., Li, J., Sun, B., & Wei, Q. (2023). Effects of Childhood Maltreatment on Self-Compassion: A Systematic Review and Meta-Analysis. *Trauma, violence & abuse*, *24*(2), 873–885. https://doi.org/10.1177/15248380211043825

3. Crego, A., Yela, J. R., Riesco-Matías, P., Gómez-Martínez, M. Á., & Vicente-Arruebarrena, A. (2022). The Benefits of Self-Compassion in Mental Health Professionals: A Systematic Review of Empirical Research. *Psychology research and behavior management*, *15*, 2599–2620. https://doi.org/10.2147/PRBM.S359382

4. Chio, F. H. N., Mak, W. W. S., & Yu, B. C. L. (2021). Meta-analytic review on the differential effects of self-compassion components on well-being and psychological distress: The moderating role of dialecticism on self-compassion. *Clinical psychology review*, *85*, 101986. https://doi.org/10.1016/j.cpr.2021.101986

5. Homan, K. J., & Sirois, F. M. (2017). Self-compassion and physical health: Exploring the roles of perceived stress and health-promoting behaviors. *Health psychology open*, *4*(2), 2055102917729542. https://doi.org/10.1177/2055102917729542

6. Winders, S. J., Murphy, O., Looney, K., & O'Reilly, G. (2020). Self-compassion, trauma, and posttraumatic stress disorder: A systematic review. *Clinical psychology & psychotherapy*, *27*(3), 300–329. https://doi.org/10.1002/cpp.2429

7. Neff K. D. (2023). Self-Compassion: Theory, Method, Research, and Intervention. *Annual review of psychology*, *74*, 193–218. https://doi.org/10.1146/annurev-psych-032420-031047

8. McDonald, M. A., Meckes, S. J., & Lancaster, C. L. (2021). Compassion for Oneself and Others Protects the Mental Health of First Responders. *Mindfulness*, *12*(3), 659–671. https://doi.org/10.1007/s12671-020-01527-y

9. Kotera, Y., Maxwell-Jones, R., Edwards, A. M., & Knutton, N. (2021). Burnout in Professional Psychotherapists: Relationships with Self-Compassion, Work-Life Balance, and Telepressure. *International journal of environmental research and public health*, *18*(10), 5308. https://doi.org/10.3390/ijerph18105308

10. Neff, K. D., & Beretvas, S. N. (2013). The role of self-compassion in romantic relationships. *Self and Identity*, *12*(1), 78–98.

11. Miyagawa, Y., & Taniguchi, J. (2022). Self-compassion helps people forgive transgressors: Cognitive pathways of interpersonal transgressions. *Self and Identity*, *21*(2), 244–256.

12. Zhang, J. W., & Chen, S. (2016). Self-Compassion Promotes Personal Improvement From Regret Experiences via Acceptance. *Personality & social psychology bulletin, 42*(2), 244–258. https://doi.org/10.1177/0146167215623271
13. Leary, M. R., Tate, E. B., Adams, C. E., Allen, A. B., & Hancock, J. (2007). Self-compassion and reactions to unpleasant self-relevant events: the implications of treating oneself kindly. *Journal of personality and social psychology, 92*(5), 887–904. https://doi.org/10.1037/0022-3514.92.5.887
14. Neff, K. (2021). Fierce Self-Compassion: How Women Can Harness Kindness to Speak Up, Claim Their Power, and Thrive. Harper.
15. Breines, J. G., & Chen, S. (2012). Self-compassion increases self-improvement motivation. *Personality & social psychology bulletin, 38*(9), 1133–1143. https://doi.org/10.1177/0146167212445599
16. Neely, M. E., Schallert, D. L., Mohammed, S. S., Roberts, R. M., & Chen, Y.-J. (2009). Self-kindness when facing stress: The role of self-compassion, goal regulation, and support in college students' well-being. *Motivation and Emotion, 33*(1), 88–97. https://doi.org/10.1007/s11031-008-9119-8
17. Hope, N., Koestner, R., & Milyavskaya, M. (2014). The role of self-compassion in goal pursuit and well-being among university freshmen. *Self and Identity, 13*(5), 579–593. https://doi.org/10.1080/15298868.2014.889032
18. Suh, H., & Chong, S. S. (2022). What Predicts Meaning in Life? The Role of Perfectionistic Personality and Self-Compassion. *Journal of Constructivist Psychology, 35*(2), 719–733. https://doi.org/10.1080/10720537.2020.1865854
19. Phillips, W. J., & Hine, D. W. (2021). Self-compassion, physical health, and health behaviour: a meta-analysis. *Health psychology review, 15*(1), 113–139. https://doi.org/10.1080/17437199.2019.1705872
20. Biber, D. D., & Ellis, R. (2019). The effect of self-compassion on the self-regulation of health behaviors: A systematic review. *Journal of health psychology, 24*(14), 2060–2071. https://doi.org/10.1177/1359105317713361
21. Sood, A. (2019). SMART with Dr. Sood. Global Center for Resiliency and Wellbeing.

25. Three Levels

1. Benuzzi, F., Lui, F., Ardizzi, M., Ambrosecchia, M., Ballotta, D., Righi, S., Pagnoni, G., Gallese, V., & Porro, C. A. (2018). Pain Mirrors: Neural Correlates of Observing Self or Others' Facial Expressions of Pain. *Frontiers in psychology, 9*, 1825. https://doi.org/10.3389/fpsyg.2018.01825
2. Beeney, J. E., Franklin, R. G., Jr, Levy, K. N., & Adams, R. B., Jr (2011). I feel your pain: emotional closeness modulates neural responses to empathically experienced rejection. *Social neuroscience, 6*(4), 369–376. https://doi.org/10.1080/17470919.2011.557245
3. Cao, Y., Contreras-Huerta, L. S., McFadyen, J., & Cunnington, R. (2015). Racial bias in neural response to others' pain is reduced with other-race contact. *Cortex; a journal devoted to the study of the nervous system and behavior, 70*, 68–78. https://doi.org/10.1016/j.cortex.2015.02.010

26. Self-Trust

1. Smirnova and J. Gatewood Owens, "Medicalized Addiction, Self-Medication, or Nonmedical Prescription Drug Use? How Trust Figures into Incarcerated Women's Conceptualization of Illicit Prescription Drug Use," Social Science & Medicine 183 (2017): 106–15, at 108.
2. Sickert, C., Klein, J. P., Altenmüller, E., & Scholz, D. S. (2022). Low Self-Esteem and Music Performance Anxiety Can Predict Depression in Musicians. *Medical problems of performing artists, 37*(4), 213–220. https://doi.org/10.21091/mppa.2022.4031
3. Joseph, B., Tseng, E. S., Zielinski, M. D., Ramirez, C. L., Lynde, J., Galey, K. M., Bhogadi, S. K., El-Qawaqzeh, K., Hosseinpour, H., & EAST Equity, Diversity, and Inclusion in Trauma Surgery Practice Committee (2023). Feeling like an imposter: are surgeons holding themselves back?. *Trauma surgery & acute care open, 8*(1), e001021. https://doi.org/10.1136/tsaco-2022-001021

4. Lee S. (2024). The effects of parental respect for children's decision-making and respect for human rights on depression in early adolescents: The mediating effect of self-esteem. *PloS one*, *19*(4), e0300320. https://doi.org/10.1371/journal.pone.0300320
5. Tottenham N. (2017). The Brain's Emotional Development. *Cerebrum : the Dana forum on brain science*, *2017*, cer-08-17.

27. Imposter Phenomenon

1. Bravata, D. M., Watts, S. A., Keefer, A. L., Madhusudhan, D. K., Taylor, K. T., Clark, D. M., Nelson, R. S., Cokley, K. O., & Hagg, H. K. (2020). Prevalence, Predictors, and Treatment of Impostor Syndrome: a Systematic Review. *Journal of general internal medicine*, *35*(4), 1252–1275. https://doi.org/10.1007/s11606-019-05364-1
2. Huecker MR, Shreffler J, McKeny PT, et al. Imposter Phenomenon. [Updated 2023 Jul 31]. In: StatPearls [Internet]. Treasure Island (FL): StatPearls Publishing; 2024 Jan-. Available from: https://www.ncbi.nlm.nih.gov/books/NBK585058/
3. Thomas, M., & Bigatti, S. (2020). Perfectionism, impostor phenomenon, and mental health in medicine: a literature review. *International journal of medical education*, *11*, 201–213. https://doi.org/10.5116/ijme.5f54.c8f8
4. Shinawatra, P., Kasirawat, C., Khunanon, P., Boonchan, S., Sangla, S., Maneeton, B., Maneeton, N., & Kawilapat, S. (2023). Exploring Factors Affecting Impostor Syndrome among Undergraduate Clinical Medical Students at Chiang Mai University, Thailand: A Cross-Sectional Study. *Behavioral sciences (Basel, Switzerland)*, *13*(12), 976. https://doi.org/10.3390/bs13120976
5. Simmons, W. K., Avery, J. A., Barcalow, J. C., Bodurka, J., Drevets, W. C., & Bellgowan, P. (2013). Keeping the body in mind: insula functional organization and functional connectivity integrate interoceptive, exteroceptive, and emotional awareness. *Human brain mapping*, *34*(11), 2944–2958. https://doi.org/10.1002/hbm.22113
6. Salminen, J. K., Saarijärvi, S., Äärelä, E., Toikka, T., & Kauhanen, J. (1999). Prevalence of alexithymia and its association with sociodemographic variables in the general population of Finland. *Journal of psychosomatic research*, *46*(1), 75–82. https://doi.org/10.1016/s0022-3999(98)00053-1
7. Bundick, M. J., Remington, K., Morton, E., & Colby, A. (2021). The contours of purpose beyond the self in midlife and later life. *Applied Developmental Science, 25*(1), 62–82. https://doi.org/10.1080/10888691.2018.1531718
8. Kobau, R., Sniezek, J., Zack, M.M., Lucas, R.E. and Burns, A. (2010), Well-Being Assessment: An Evaluation of Well-Being Scales for Public Health and Population Estimates of Well-Being among US Adults. Applied Psychology: Health and Well-Being, 2: 272-297. https://doi.org/10.1111/j.1758-0854.2010.01035.x
9. Beck ED, Yoneda T, James BD, et al. Personality predictors of dementia diagnosis and neuropathological burden: An individual participant data meta-analysis. *Alzheimer's Dement*. 2024; 20: 1497–1514. https://doi.org/10.1002/alz.13523
10. Bock, M. A., Bahorik, A., Brenowitz, W. D., & Yaffe, K. (2020). Apathy and risk of probable incident dementia among community-dwelling older adults. *Neurology*, *95*(24), e3280–e3287. https://doi.org/10.1212/WNL.0000000000010951
11. Johnson, R., Grove, A., & Clarke, A. (2018). It's hard to play ball: A qualitative study of knowledge exchange and silo effects in public health. *BMC health services research*, *18*(1), 1. https://doi.org/10.1186/s12913-017-2770-6
12. Håkanson, Cecilia PhD, RN. Everyday Life, Healthcare, and Self-Care Management Among People With Irritable Bowel Syndrome: An Integrative Review of Qualitative Research. Gastroenterology Nursing 37(3):p 217-225, May/June 2014. | DOI: 10.1097/SGA.0000000000000048

28. Actionable Insights

1. Reddan, M. C., Wager, T. D., & Schiller, D. (2018). Attenuating Neural Threat Expression with Imagination. *Neuron*, *100*(4), 994–1005.e4. https://doi.org/10.1016/j.neuron.2018.10.047

29. Self-Compassion Practices

1. Sarmiento, L. F., Lopes da Cunha, P., Tabares, S., Tafet, G., & Gouveia, A., Jr (2024). Decision-making under stress: A psychological and neurobiological integrative model. *Brain, behavior, & immunity - health*, *38*, 100766. https://doi.org/10.1016/j.bbih.2024.100766
2. Arnsten A. F. (2015). Stress weakens prefrontal networks: molecular insults to higher cognition. *Nature neuroscience*, *18*(10), 1376–1385. https://doi.org/10.1038/nn.4087
3. Woo, E., Sansing, L. H., Arnsten, A. F. T., & Datta, D. (2021). Chronic Stress Weakens Connectivity in the Prefrontal Cortex: Architectural and Molecular Changes. *Chronic stress (Thousand Oaks, Calif.)*, *5*, 24705470211029254. https://doi.org/10.1177/24705470211029254
4. Zaccaro, A., Piarulli, A., Laurino, M., Garbella, E., Menicucci, D., Neri, B., & Gemignani, A. (2018). How Breath-Control Can Change Your Life: A Systematic Review on Psycho-Physiological Correlates of Slow Breathing. *Frontiers in human neuroscience*, *12*, 353. https://doi.org/10.3389/fnhum.2018.00353
5. Steele, C. M. (1988). The psychology of self-affirmation: Sustaining the integrity of the self. In L. Berkowitz (Ed.), *Advances in experimental social psychology, Vol. 21. Social psychological studies of the self: Perspectives and programs* (pp. 261–302). Academic Press.
6. Hirosaki, M., Ohira, T., Wu, Y., Eguchi, E., Shirai, K., Imano, H., Funakubo, N., Nishizawa, H., Katakami, N., Shimomura, I., & Iso, H. (2023). Laughter yoga as an enjoyable therapeutic approach for glycemic control in individuals with type 2 diabetes: A randomized controlled trial. *Frontiers in endocrinology*, *14*, 1148468.
7. Öztürk, F. Ö., Bayraktar, E. P., & Tezel, A. (2023). The effect of laughter yoga on loneliness, psychological resilience, and quality of life in older adults: A pilot randomized controlled trial. *Geriatric nursing (New York, N.Y.)*, *50*, 208–214. https://doi.org/10.1016/j.gerinurse.2023.01.009
8. Bressington, D., Mui, J., Yu, C., Leung, S. F., Cheung, K., Wu, C. S. T., Bollard, M., & Chien, W. T. (2019). Feasibility of a group-based laughter yoga intervention as an adjunctive treatment for residual symptoms of depression, anxiety and stress in people with depression. *Journal of affective disorders*, *248*, 42–51.
9. Stark, S., Stark, C., Wong, B., & Brin, M. F. (2023). Modulation of amygdala activity for emotional faces due to botulinum toxin type A injections that prevent frowning. *Scientific reports*, *13*(1), 3333. https://doi.org/10.1038/s41598-023-29280-x
10. Alam, M., Barrett, K. C., Hodapp, R. M., & Arndt, K. A. (2008). Botulinum toxin and the facial feedback hypothesis: can looking better make you feel happier?. *Journal of the American Academy of Dermatology*, *58*(6), 1061–1072. https://doi.org/10.1016/j.jaad.2007.10.649
11. Stark, S., Stark, C., Wong, B., & Brin, M. F. (2023). Modulation of amygdala activity for emotional faces due to botulinum toxin type A injections that prevent frowning. *Scientific reports*, *13*(1), 3333. https://doi.org/10.1038/s41598-023-29280-x
12. Alam, M., Barrett, K. C., Hodapp, R. M., & Arndt, K. A. (2008). Botulinum toxin and the facial feedback hypothesis: can looking better make you feel happier?. *Journal of the American Academy of Dermatology*, *58*(6), 1061–1072. https://doi.org/10.1016/j.jaad.2007.10.649
13. Finzi E. (2023). Botulinum Toxin Treatment for Depression: A New Paradigm for Psychiatry. *Toxins*, *15*(5), 336. https://doi.org/10.3390/toxins15050336
14. Demchenko, I., Swiderski, A., Liu, H., Jung, H., Lou, W., & Bhat, V. (2024). Botulinum Toxin Injections for Psychiatric Disorders: A Systematic Review of the Clinical Trial Landscape. *Toxins*, *16*(4), 191. https://doi.org/10.3390/toxins16040191
15. Creswell, J. D., Welch, W. T., Taylor, S. E., Sherman, D. K., Gruenewald, T. L., & Mann, T. (2005). Affirmation of personal values buffers neuroendocrine and psychological stress responses. *Psychological science*, *16*(11), 846–851. https://doi.org/10.1111/j.1467-9280.2005.01624.x
16. Creswell, J. D., Dutcher, J. M., Klein, W. M., Harris, P. R., & Levine, J. M. (2013). Self-affirmation improves problem-solving under stress. *PloS one*, *8*(5), e62593. https://doi.org/10.1371/journal.pone.0062593

17. Yildirim, M., Akbal, S., & Turkoglu, M. (2023). The effect of self-affirmation on anxiety and perceived discomfort in patients who have undergone open-heart surgery. A randomized controlled trial. *Applied nursing research : ANR, 72*, 151687. https://doi.org/10.1016/j.apnr.2023.151687
18. Logel, C., & Cohen, G. L. (2012). The role of the self in physical health: testing the effect of a values-affirmation intervention on weight loss. *Psychological science, 23*(1), 53–55. https://doi.org/10.1177/0956797611421936
19. Wileman, V., Farrington, K., Chilcot, J., Norton, S., Wellsted, D. M., Almond, M. K., Davenport, A., Franklin, G., Gane, M.daS., & Armitage, C. J. (2014). Evidence that self-affirmation improves phosphate control in hemodialysis patients: a pilot cluster randomized controlled trial. *Annals of behavioral medicine : a publication of the Society of Behavioral Medicine, 48*(2), 275–281. https://doi.org/10.1007/s12160-014-9597-8
20. Cohen, G. L., Garcia, J., Apfel, N., & Master, A. (2006). Reducing the racial achievement gap: a social-psychological intervention. *Science (New York, N.Y.), 313*(5791), 1307–1310. https://doi.org/10.1126/science.1128317
21. Hadden, I. R., Easterbrook, M. J., Nieuwenhuis, M., Fox, K. J., & Dolan, P. (2020). Self-affirmation reduces the socioeconomic attainment gap in schools in England. *The British journal of educational psychology, 90*(2), 517–536. https://doi.org/10.1111/bjep.12291
22. Cascio, C. N., O'Donnell, M. B., Tinney, F. J., Lieberman, M. D., Taylor, S. E., Strecher, V. J., & Falk, E. B. (2016). Self-affirmation activates brain systems associated with self-related processing and reward and is reinforced by future orientation. *Social cognitive and affective neuroscience, 11*(4), 621–629. https://doi.org/10.1093/scan/nsv136
23. Tisdell, E. J., Lukic, B., Banerjee, R., Liao, D., & Palmer, C. (2024). The Effects of Heart Rhythm Meditation on Vagal Tone and Well-being: A Mixed Methods Research Study. *Applied psychophysiology and biofeedback*, 10.1007/s10484-024-09639-0. Advance online publication. https://doi.org/10.1007/s10484-024-09639-0
24. Tee, V., Kuan, G., Kueh, Y. C., Abdullah, N., Sabran, K., Tagiling, N., Sahran, N. F., Alang, T. A. I. T., & Lee, Y. Y. (2022). Development and validation of audio-based guided imagery and progressive muscle relaxation tools for functional bloating. *PloS one, 17*(9), e0268491. https://doi.org/10.1371/journal.pone.0268491
25. Colzato, L. S., Ritter, S. M., & Steenbergen, L. (2018). Transcutaneous vagus nerve stimulation (tVNS) enhances divergent thinking. *Neuropsychologia, 111*, 72–76. https://doi.org/10.1016/j.neuropsychologia.2018.01.003
26. Colzato, L., & Beste, C. (2020). A literature review on the neurophysiological underpinnings and cognitive effects of transcutaneous vagus nerve stimulation: challenges and future directions. *Journal of neurophysiology, 123*(5), 1739–1755. https://doi.org/10.1152/jn.00057.2020
27. Álvarez-García, C., & Yaban, Z. Ş. (2020). The effects of preoperative guided imagery interventions on preoperative anxiety and postoperative pain: A meta-analysis. *Complementary therapies in clinical practice, 38*, 101077. https://doi.org/10.1016/j.ctcp.2019.101077
28. Vagnoli, L., Bettini, A., Amore, E., De Masi, S., & Messeri, A. (2019). Relaxation-guided imagery reduces perioperative anxiety and pain in children: a randomized study. *European journal of pediatrics, 178*(6), 913–921. https://doi.org/10.1007/s00431-019-03376-x
29. Zemla, K., Sedek, G., Wróbel, K., Postepski, F., & Wojcik, G. M. (2023). Investigating the Impact of Guided Imagery on Stress, Brain Functions, and Attention: A Randomized Trial. *Sensors (Basel, Switzerland), 23*(13), 6210. https://doi.org/10.3390/s23136210
30. Giacobbi, P., Jr, Long, D., Nolan, R., Shawley, S., Johnson, K., & Misra, R. (2018). Guided imagery targeting exercise, food cravings, and stress: a multi-modal randomized feasibility trial. *Journal of behavioral medicine, 41*(1), 87–98. https://doi.org/10.1007/s10865-017-9876-5
31. Charalambous, A., Giannakopoulou, M., Bozas, E., Marcou, Y., Kitsios, P., & Paikousis, L. (2016). Guided Imagery And Progressive Muscle Relaxation as a Cluster of Symptoms Management Intervention in Patients Receiving Chemotherapy: A Randomized Control Trial. *PloS one, 11*(6), e0156911. https://doi.org/10.1371/journal.pone.0156911

32. Giacobbi, P., Jr, Long, D., Nolan, R., Shawley, S., Johnson, K., & Misra, R. (2018). Guided imagery targeting exercise, food cravings, and stress: a multi-modal randomized feasibility trial. *Journal of behavioral medicine*, *41*(1), 87–98. https://doi.org/10.1007/s10865-017-9876-5

33. Zech, N., Hansen, E., Bernardy, K., & Häuser, W. (2017). Efficacy, acceptability and safety of guided imagery/hypnosis in fibromyalgia - A systematic review and meta-analysis of randomized controlled trials. *European journal of pain (London, England)*, *21*(2), 217–227. https://doi.org/10.1002/ejp.933

34. Hadjibalassi, M., Lambrinou, E., Papastavrou, E., & Papathanassoglou, E. (2018). The effect of guided imagery on physiological and psychological outcomes of adult ICU patients: A systematic literature review and methodological implications. *Australian critical care : official journal of the Confederation of Australian Critical Care Nurses*, *31*(2), 73–86. https://doi.org/10.1016/j.aucc.2017.03.001

35. Kantola, M., Ilves, O., Honkanen, S., Hakonen, H., Yli-Ikkelä, R., Köyhäjoki, A., Anttila, M. R., Rintala, A., Korpi, H., Sjögren, T., Karvanen, J., & Aartolahti, E. (2024). The Effects of Virtual Reality Training on Cognition in Older Adults: A Systematic Review, Meta-Analysis, and Meta-Regression of Randomized Controlled Trials. *Journal of aging and physical activity*, *32*(3), 321–349. https://doi.org/10.1123/japa.2023-0217

36. Baradwan, S., Alshahrani, M. S., AlSghan, R., Alyafi, M., Elsayed, R. E., Abdel-Hakam, F. A., Moustafa, A. A., Hussien, A. E., Yahia, O. S., Shama, A. A., Magdy, A. A., Abdelhakim, A. M., & Badran, H. (2024). The effect of virtual reality on pain and anxiety management during outpatient hysteroscopy: a systematic review and meta-analysis of randomized controlled trials. *Archives of gynecology and obstetrics*, *309*(4), 1267–1280. https://doi.org/10.1007/s00404-023-07319-8

37. Li, R., Li, Y., Kong, Y., Li, H., Hu, D., Fu, C., & Wei, Q. (2024). Virtual Reality-Based Training in Chronic Low Back Pain: Systematic Review and Meta-Analysis of Randomized Controlled Trials. *Journal of medical Internet research*, *26*, e45406. https://doi.org/10.2196/45406

38. Blázquez-González, P., Mirón-González, R., Lendínez-Mesa, A., Luengo-González, R., Mancebo-Salas, N., Camacho-Arroyo, M. T., & Martínez-Hortelano, J. A. (2024). Impact of virtual reality-based therapy on post-stroke depression: A systematic review and meta-analysis of randomized controlled trials. *Worldviews on evidence-based nursing*, *21*(2), 194–201. https://doi.org/10.1111/wvn.12699

39. Rejbrand, C., Fure, B., & Sonnby, K. (2023). Stand-alone virtual reality exposure therapy as a treatment for social anxiety symptoms: a systematic review and meta-analysis. *Upsala journal of medical sciences*, *128*, 10.48101/ujms.v128.9289. https://doi.org/10.48101/ujms.v128.9289

40. Lee, J., Phu, S., Lord, S. R., & Okubo, Y. (2024). Effects of immersive virtual reality training on balance, gait and mobility in older adults: A systematic review and meta-analysis. *Gait & posture*, *110*, 129–137. https://doi.org/10.1016/j.gaitpost.2024.03.009

41. Park, S., Chung, C., & Kim, G. (2023). Effects of Health Education Using Virtual Reality for Adolescents: A Systematic Review and Meta-Analysis. *Journal of Korean Academy of Nursing*, *53*(2), 177–190. https://doi.org/10.4040/jkan.23003

42. Weissman D. E. (2011). Martyrs in palliative care. *Journal of palliative medicine*, *14*(12), 1278–1279. https://doi.org/10.1089/jpm.2011.0293

43. Macauley, R., Elster, N., Fanaroff, J. M., & COMMITTEE ON BIOETHICS, COMMITTEE ON MEDICAL LIABILITY AND RISK MANAGEMENT (2021). Ethical Considerations in Pediatricians' Use of Social Media. *Pediatrics*, *147*(3), e2020049685. https://doi.org/10.1542/peds.2020-049685

44. *APA Dictionary of Psychology*. APA, 2023. https://dictionary.apa.org/

45. Mammoliti M: *Why Boundaries Should be Part of Your 2022 Physician Goals: Medpage Today*, 2022. https://www.kevinmd.com/2022/02/why-boundaries-should-be-part-of-your-2022-physician-goals.html

46. Chatwal, M. S., Kamal, A. H., & Marron, J. M. (2023). Fear of Saying No (FOSNO): Setting Boundaries With Our Patients and Ourselves. *American Society of Clinical Oncology educational book. American Society of Clinical Oncology. Annual Meeting*, *43*, e390598. https://doi.org/10.1200/EDBK_390598

47. Nadkarni, A., Behbahani, K., & Fromson, J. (2023). When Compromised Professional Fulfillment Compromises Professionalism. *JAMA*, *329*(14), 1147–1148. https://doi.org/10.1001/jama.2023.2076

48. Firth, J., Gangwisch, J. E., Borisini, A., Wootton, R. E., & Mayer, E. A. (2020). Food and mood: how do diet and nutrition affect mental wellbeing?. *BMJ (Clinical research ed.)*, *369*, m2382. https://doi.org/10.1136/bmj.m2382

49. Mujcic, R., & J Oswald, A. (2016). Evolution of Well-Being and Happiness After Increases in Consumption of Fruit and Vegetables. *American journal of public health*, *106*(8), 1504–1510. https://doi.org/10.2105/AJPH.2016.303260

50. Metzler, H., Vilarem, E., Petschen, A., & Grèzes, J. (2023). Power pose effects on approach and avoidance decisions in response to social threat. *PloS one*, *18*(8), e0286904. https://doi.org/10.1371/journal.pone.0286904

51. Cuddy, A. J. C., Wilmuth, C. A., Yap, A. J., & Carney, D. R. (2015). Preparatory power posing affects nonverbal presence and job interview performance. *The Journal of applied psychology*, *100*(4), 1286–1295. https://doi.org/10.1037/a0038543

52. Davis, M. L., Papini, S., Rosenfield, D., Roelofs, K., Kolb, S., Powers, M. B., & Smits, J. A. J. (2017). A randomized controlled study of power posing before public speaking exposure for social anxiety disorder: No evidence for augmentative effects. *Journal of anxiety disorders*, *52*, 1–7. https://doi.org/10.1016/j.janxdis.2017.09.004

53. Slater, D., Korakakis, V., O'Sullivan, P., Nolan, D., & O'Sullivan, K. (2019). "Sit Up Straight": Time to Re-evaluate. *The Journal of orthopaedic and sports physical therapy*, *49*(8), 562–564. https://doi.org/10.2519/jospt.2019.0610

54. O'Sullivan, K., O'Sullivan, P., O'Sullivan, L., & Dankaerts, W. (2012). What do physiotherapists consider to be the best sitting spinal posture?. *Manual therapy*, *17*(5), 432–437. https://doi.org/10.1016/j.math.2012.04.007

55. https://medlineplus.gov/guidetogoodposture.html#

56. Korakakis, V., O'Sullivan, K., O'Sullivan, P. B., Evagelinou, V., Sotiralis, Y., Sideris, A., Sakellariou, K., Karanasios, S., & Giakas, G. (2019). Physiotherapist perceptions of optimal sitting and standing posture. *Musculoskeletal science & practice*, *39*, 24–31. https://doi.org/10.1016/j.msksp.2018.11.004

57. Smythe, A., & Jivanjee, M. (2021). The straight and narrow of posture: Current clinical concepts. *Australian journal of general practice*, *50*(11), 807–810. https://doi.org/10.31128/AJGP-07-21-6083

58. Nair, S., Sagar, M., Sollers, J., 3rd, Consedine, N., & Broadbent, E. (2015). Do slumped and upright postures affect stress responses? A randomized trial. *Health psychology : official journal of the Division of Health Psychology, American Psychological Association*, *34*(6), 632–641. https://doi.org/10.1037/hea0000146

59. Wilkes, C., Kydd, R., Sagar, M., & Broadbent, E. (2017). Upright posture improves affect and fatigue in people with depressive symptoms. *Journal of behavior therapy and experimental psychiatry*, *54*, 143–149. https://doi.org/10.1016/j.jbtep.2016.07.015

60. Hackford, J., Mackey, A., & Broadbent, E. (2019). The effects of walking posture on affective and physiological states during stress. *Journal of behavior therapy and experimental psychiatry*, *62*, 80–87. https://doi.org/10.1016/j.jbtep.2018.09.004

61. Sherman, L. E., Hernandez, L. M., Greenfield, P. M., & Dapretto, M. (2018). What the brain 'Likes': neural correlates of providing feedback on social media. *Social cognitive and affective neuroscience*, *13*(7), 699–707. https://doi.org/10.1093/scan/nsy051

62. Sherman, L. E., Payton, A. A., Hernandez, L. M., Greenfield, P. M., & Dapretto, M. (2016). The Power of the Like in Adolescence: Effects of Peer Influence on Neural and Behavioral Responses to Social Media. *Psychological science*, *27*(7), 1027–1035. https://doi.org/10.1177/0956797616645673

63. Domínguez D, J. F., Taing, S. A., & Molenberghs, P. (2016). Why Do Some Find it Hard to Disagree? An fMRI Study. *Frontiers in human neuroscience*, *9*, 718. https://doi.org/10.3389/fnhum.2015.00718

64. Chevalier, G., Sinatra, S. T., Oschman, J. L., Sokal, K., & Sokal, P. (2012). Earthing: health implications of reconnecting the human body to the Earth's surface electrons. *Journal of environmental and public health*, *2012*, 291541. https://doi.org/10.1155/2012/291541

65. Sinatra, S. T., Oschman, J. L., Chevalier, G., & Sinatra, D. (2017). Electric Nutrition: The Surprising Health and Healing Benefits of Biological Grounding (Earthing). *Alternative therapies in health and medicine*, *23*(5), 8–16.

66. Oschman, J. L., Chevalier, G., & Brown, R. (2015). The effects of grounding (earthing) on inflammation, the immune response, wound healing, and prevention and treatment of chronic inflammatory and autoimmune diseases. *Journal of inflammation research*, *8*, 83–96. https://doi.org/10.2147/JIR.S69656

67. Chevalier, G., Sinatra, S. T., Oschman, J. L., & Delany, R. M. (2013). Earthing (grounding) the human body reduces blood viscosity-a major factor in cardiovascular disease. *Journal of alternative and complementary medicine (New York, N.Y.)*, *19*(2), 102–110. https://doi.org/10.1089/acm.2011.0820

68. Chevalier, G., Patel, S., Weiss, L., Chopra, D., & Mills, P. J. (2019). The Effects of Grounding (Earthing) on Bodyworkers' Pain and Overall Quality of Life: A Randomized Controlled Trial. *Explore (New York, N.Y.)*, *15*(3), 181–190. https://doi.org/10.1016/j.explore.2018.10.001

69. Menigoz, W., Latz, T. T., Ely, R. A., Kamei, C., Melvin, G., & Sinatra, D. (2020). Integrative and lifestyle medicine strategies should include Earthing (grounding): Review of research evidence and clinical observations. *Explore (New York, N.Y.)*, *16*(3), 152–160. https://doi.org/10.1016/j.explore.2019.10.005

70. Jamieson I. A. (2023). Grounding (earthing) as related to electromagnetic hygiene: An integrative review. *Biomedical journal*, *46*(1), 30–40. https://doi.org/10.1016/j.bj.2022.11.005

71. Stillman, P. E., Van Bavel, J. J., & Cunningham, W. A. (2015). Valence asymmetries in the human amygdala: task relevance modulates amygdala responses to positive more than negative affective cues. *Journal of cognitive neuroscience*, *27*(4), 842–851. https://doi.org/10.1162/jocn_a_00756

72. Cunningham, W. A., & Kirkland, T. (2014). The joyful, yet balanced, amygdala: moderated responses to positive but not negative stimuli in trait happiness. *Social cognitive and affective neuroscience*, *9*(6), 760–766. https://doi.org/10.1093/scan/nst045

73. Roche, K., Mulchan, S., Ayr-Volta, L., Elias, M., Brimacombe, M., Morello, C., & Hinderer, K. A. (2023). Pilot Study on the Impact of Gratitude Journaling or Cognitive Strategies on Health Care Workers. *Journal of pediatric health care : official publication of National Association of Pediatric Nurse Associates & Practitioners*, *37*(4), 414–424. https://doi.org/10.1016/j.pedhc.2023.02.002

74. Ricker, M., Brooks, A. J., Bodine, S., Lebensohn, P., & Maizes, V. (2021). Well-being in Residency: Impact of an Online Physician Well-being Course on Resiliency and Burnout in Incoming Residents. *Family medicine*, *53*(2), 123–128. https://doi.org/10.22454/FamMed.2021.314886

75. Nawa, N. E., & Yamagishi, N. (2021). Enhanced academic motivation in university students following a 2-week online gratitude journal intervention. *BMC psychology*, *9*(1), 71. https://doi.org/10.1186/s40359-021-00559-w

76. King, R. B., & Datu, J. A. D. (2018). Grateful students are motivated, engaged, and successful in school: Cross-sectional, longitudinal, and experimental evidence. *Journal of school psychology*, *70*, 105–122. https://doi.org/10.1016/j.jsp.2018.08.001

77. Cook, K. A., Woessner, K. M., & White, A. A. (2018). Happy asthma: Improved asthma control with a gratitude journal. *The journal of allergy and clinical immunology. In practice*, *6*(6), 2154–2156. https://doi.org/10.1016/j.jaip.2018.04.021

78. McGinness, A., Raman, M., Stallworth, D., & Natesan, S. (2022). App-Based Three Good Things and Gratitude Journaling Incentive Program for Burnout in Pediatric Residents: A Nonrandomized Controlled Pilot. *Academic pediatrics*, *22*(8), 1532–1535. https://doi.org/10.1016/j.acap.2022.05.009

79. Field T. (2016). Massage therapy research review. *Complementary therapies in clinical practice*, *24*, 19–31. https://doi.org/10.1016/j.ctcp.2016.04.005

80. Chetry, D., Telles, S., & Balkrishna, A. (2021). A PubMed-Based Exploration of the Course of Yoga Research from 1948 to 2020. *International journal of yoga therapy*, *31*(1), Article_22. https://doi.org/10.17761/2021-D-21-00017

81. Daviet, R., Aydogan, G., Jagannathan, K., Spilka, N., Koellinger, P. D., Kranzler, H. R., Nave, G., & Wetherill, R. R. (2022). Associations between alcohol consumption and gray and white matter

volumes in the UK Biobank. *Nature communications*, *13*(1), 1175. https://doi.org/10.1038/s41467-022-28735-5

30. Eight Billion Sages

31. What is Self-acceptance?
1. BYRNE D. (1961). Interpersonal attraction and attitude similarity. *Journal of abnormal and social psychology*, *62*, 713–715. https://doi.org/10.1037/h0044721
2. Montoya R. M., Horton R. S., Kirchner J. (2008). Is actual similarity necessary for attraction? A meta-analysis of actual and perceived similarity. *J. Soc. Pers. Relationsh.* 25 889–922.
3. Krypotos, A. M., Effting, M., Kindt, M., & Beckers, T. (2015). Avoidance learning: a review of theoretical models and recent developments. *Frontiers in behavioral neuroscience*, *9*, 189. https://doi.org/10.3389/fnbeh.2015.00189
4. Cancino-Montecinos, S., Björklund, F., & Lindholm, T. (2020). A General Model of Dissonance Reduction: Unifying Past Accounts via an Emotion Regulation Perspective. *Frontiers in psychology*, *11*, 540081. https://doi.org/10.3389/fpsyg.2020.540081
5. Festinger, L. (1957). *A theory of cognitive dissonance*. Evanston, IL: Row, Peterson and Company.

32. Self-acceptance: Why
1. Key Substance Use and Mental Health Indicators in the United States: Results from the 2022 National Survey on Drug Use and Health. Substance Abuse and Mental Health Services Administration. Accessed 7/24/2024.
2. Mental Health By the Numbers. National Alliance on Mental Health. Accessed 7/24/2024.
3. Mental Illness. National Institute of Mental Health. Accessed 7/24/2024.
4. Facts About Suicide. Centers for Disease Control and Prevention. Accessed 7/24/2024.
5. Suicide. National Institute of Mental Health. Accessed 7/24/2024.
6. The State of Mental Health in America. Mental Health America. Accessed 7/24/2023.
7. O'Súilleabháin, P. S., D'Arcy-Bewick, S., Fredrix, M., McGeehan, M., Kirwan, E., Willard, M., Sesker, A. A., Sutin, A. R., & Turiano, N. A. (2024). Self-Acceptance and Purpose in Life Are Mechanisms Linking Adverse Childhood Experiences to Mortality Risk. *Psychosomatic medicine*, *86*(2), 83–88. https://doi.org/10.1097/PSY.0000000000001266
8. Sanghvi, D. E., Zainal, N. H., & Newman, M. G. (2023). Trait self-acceptance mediates parental childhood abuse predicting depression and anxiety symptoms in adulthood. *Journal of anxiety disorders*, *94*, 102673. https://doi.org/10.1016/j.janxdis.2023.102673
9. Hawes, T., Zimmer-Gembeck, M. J., & Campbell, S. M. (2020). Unique associations of social media use and online appearance preoccupation with depression, anxiety, and appearance rejection sensitivity. *Body image*, *33*, 66–76. https://doi.org/10.1016/j.bodyim.2020.02.010
10. Jarman, H. K., Marques, M. D., McLean, S. A., Slater, A., & Paxton, S. J. (2021). Social media, body satisfaction and well-being among adolescents: A mediation model of appearance-ideal internalization and comparison. *Body image*, *36*, 139–148. https://doi.org/10.1016/j.bodyim.2020.11.005
11. Markey, C. H., & Daniels, E. A. (2022). An examination of preadolescent girls' social media use and body image: Type of engagement may matter most. *Body image*, *42*, 145–149. https://doi.org/10.1016/j.bodyim.2022.05.005
12. Fardouly, J., Magson, N. R., Rapee, R. M., Johnco, C. J., & Oar, E. L. (2020). The use of social media by Australian preadolescents and its links with mental health. *Journal of clinical psychology*, *76*(7), 1304–1326. https://doi.org/10.1002/jclp.22936
13. Ruan, Q. N., Shen, G. H., Yang, J. S., & Yan, W. J. (2023). The interplay of self-acceptance, social comparison and attributional style in adolescent mental health: cross-sectional study. *BJPsych open*, *9*(6), e202. https://doi.org/10.1192/bjo.2023.594

14. Yang, Q., Xu, Y., & van den Bos, K. (2024). Social network site use and materialistic values: the roles of self-control and self-acceptance. *BMC psychology*, *12*(1), 55. https://doi.org/10.1186/s40359-024-01546-7

15. Kong, L., Gao, Z., Xu, N., Shao, S., Ma, H., He, Q., Zhang, D., Xu, H., & Qu, H. (2021). The relation between self-stigma and loneliness in visually impaired college students: Self-acceptance as mediator. *Disability and health journal*, *14*(2), 101054. https://doi.org/10.1016/j.dhjo.2020.101054

16. Crapolicchio, E., Vezzali, L., & Regalia, C. (2021). "I forgive myself": The association between self-criticism, self-acceptance, and PTSD in women victims of IPV, and the buffering role of self-efficacy. *Journal of community psychology*, *49*(2), 252–265. https://doi.org/10.1002/jcop.22454

17. De Nardo, T., Gabel, R. M., Tetnowski, J. A., & Swartz, E. R. (2016). Self-acceptance of stuttering: A preliminary study. *Journal of communication disorders*, *60*, 27–38. https://doi.org/10.1016/j.jcomdis.2016.02.003

18. Joshanloo M. (2022). The Temporal Relationship Between Self-Acceptance and Generativity over Two Decades. *Journal of applied gerontology : the official journal of the Southern Gerontological Society*, *41*(3), 842–846. https://doi.org/10.1177/07334648211061476

19. Li, S., Zhang, X., Luo, C., Chen, M., Xie, X., Gong, F., Lv, F., Xu, J., Han, J., Fu, L., & Sun, Y. (2021). The mediating role of self-acceptance in the relationship between loneliness and subjective well-being among the elderly in nursing home: A cross-sectional study. *Medicine*, *100*(40), e27364. https://doi.org/10.1097/MD.0000000000027364

20. Ng, R., Allore, H. G., & Levy, B. R. (2020). Self-Acceptance and Interdependence Promote Longevity: Evidence From a 20-year Prospective Cohort Study. *International journal of environmental research and public health*, *17*(16), 5980. https://doi.org/10.3390/ijerph17165980

21. Messina, I., Grecucci, A., & Viviani, R. (2021). Neurobiological models of emotion regulation: a meta-analysis of neuroimaging studies of acceptance as an emotion regulation strategy. *Social cognitive and affective neuroscience*, *16*(3), 257–267. https://doi.org/10.1093/scan/nsab007

33. Self-acceptance: How (Insights)

1. Uğur, E., Kaya, Ç., & Tanhan, A. (2021). Psychological inflexibility mediates the relationship between fear of negative evaluation and psychological vulnerability. *Current psychology (New Brunswick, N.J.)*, *40*(9), 4265–4277. https://doi.org/10.1007/s12144-020-01074-8; Pyszkowska, A., & Rönnlund, M. (2021). Psychological Flexibility and Self-Compassion as Predictors of Well-Being: Mediating Role of a Balanced Time Perspective. *Frontiers in psychology*, *12*, 671746. https://doi.org/10.3389/fpsyg.2021.671746

2. Ferradás, M. D. M., Freire, C., Núñez, J. C., & Regueiro, B. (2019). Associations between Profiles of Self-Esteem and Achievement Goals and the Protection of Self-Worth in University Students. *International journal of environmental research and public health*, *16*(12), 2218. https://doi.org/10.3390/ijerph16122218

3. Osaji, J., Ojimba, C., & Ahmed, S. (2020). The Use of Acceptance and Commitment Therapy in Substance Use Disorders: A Review of Literature. *Journal of clinical medicine research*, *12*(10), 629–633. https://doi.org/10.14740/jocmr4311; Alavi H. R. (2011). The Role of Self-esteem in Tendency towards Drugs, Theft and Prostitution. *Addiction & health*, *3*(3-4), 119–124.

34. Self-acceptance: How (Practices)

1. Qian, Y., Yu, X., & Liu, F. (2022). Comparison of Two Approaches to Enhance Self-Esteem and Self-Acceptance in Chinese College Students: Psychoeducational Lecture vs. Group Intervention. *Frontiers in psychology*, *13*, 877737. https://doi.org/10.3389/fpsyg.2022.877737

2. Briganti, G., Fried, E. I., & Linkowski, P. (2019). Network analysis of Contingencies of Self-Worth Scale in 680 university students. *Psychiatry research*, *272*, 252–257. https://doi.org/10.1016/j.psychres.2018.12.080

3. Steele, C. M. (1988). The psychology of self-affirmation: Sustaining the integrity of the self. In L. Berkowitz (Ed.), *Advances in experimental social psychology, Vol. 21. Social psychological studies of the self: Perspectives and programs* (pp. 261–302). Academic Press.

4. Sherman D.K., Cohen G.L. (2006). The psychology of self-defense: self-affirmation theory. *Advances in Experimental Social Psychology*, 38, 183.
5. Cohen G.L., Sherman D.K. (2014). The psychology of change: self-affirmation and social psychological intervention. *Annual Review of Psychology*, 65, 333–71
6. Schacter D.L. (2012). Adaptive constructive processes and the future of memory. *American Psychologist*, 67(8), 603.
7. Benoit R.G., Schacter D.L. (2015). Specifying the core network supporting episodic simulation and episodic memory by activation likelihood estimation. *Neuropsychologia*, 75, 450–7.
8. Cascio, C. N., O'Donnell, M. B., Tinney, F. J., Lieberman, M. D., Taylor, S. E., Strecher, V. J., & Falk, E. B. (2016). Self-affirmation activates brain systems associated with self-related processing and reward and is reinforced by future orientation. *Social cognitive and affective neuroscience*, *11*(4), 621–629. https://doi.org/10.1093/scan/nsv136
9. Seligman, M.E.P. Railton, P., Baumeister, R.F., & Sripada, C. (2016). Homo Prospectus. Oxford University Press.
10. Creswell, J. D., Welch, W. T., Taylor, S. E., Sherman, D. K., Gruenewald, T. L., & Mann, T. (2005). Affirmation of personal values buffers neuroendocrine and psychological stress responses. Psychological Science, 16(11), 846-851
11. Creswell, J. D., Dutcher, J. M., Klein, W. M., Harris, P. R., & Levine, J. M. (2013). Self-affirmation improves problem-solving under stress. PLoS ONE, 8(5), e62593
12. Sherman, D. K., Bunyan, D. P., Creswell, J. D., & Jaremka, L. M. (2009). Psychological vulnerability and stress: the effects of self-affirmation on sympathetic nervous system responses to naturalistic stressors. Health Psychology, 28(5), 554
13. Lamont M. (2019). From 'having' to 'being': self-worth and the current crisis of American society. *The British journal of sociology*, *70*(3), 660–707. https://doi.org/10.1111/1468-4446.12667
14. Ravary, A., Stewart, E. K., & Baldwin, M. W. (2020). Insecurity about getting old: age-contingent self-worth, attentional bias, and well-being. *Aging & mental health*, *24*(10), 1636–1644. https://doi.org/10.1080/13607863.2019.1636202
15. Frey, W. H., 2nd, DeSota-Johnson, D., Hoffman, C., & McCall, J. T. (1981). Effect of stimulus on the chemical composition of human tears. *American journal of ophthalmology*, *92*(4), 559–567. https://doi.org/10.1016/0002-9394(81)90651-6
16. Kuyumcu, B., & Rohner, R. P. (2018). The relation between remembered parental acceptance in childhood and self-acceptance among young Turkish adults. *International journal of psychology : Journal international de psychologie*, *53*(2), 126–132. https://doi.org/10.1002/ijop.12277
17. Sood, A. (2019). SMART with Dr. Sood. Global Center for Resiliency and Wellbeing.
18. Lieberman, M. D., Eisenberger, N. I., Crockett, M. J., Tom, S. M., Pfeifer, J. H., & Way, B. M. (2007). Putting feelings into words: affect labeling disrupts amygdala activity in response to affective stimuli. *Psychological science*, *18*(5), 421–428. https://doi.org/10.1111/j.1467-9280.2007.01916.x

35. This You Know Already

1. Billingsley, J., & Losin, E. A. R. (2017). The Neural Systems of Forgiveness: An Evolutionary Psychological Perspective. *Frontiers in psychology*, *8*, 737. https://doi.org/10.3389/fpsyg.2017.00737
2. Li, H., Wang, W., Li, J., Qiu, J., & Wu, Y. (2024). Spontaneous brain activity associated with individual differences in decisional and emotional forgiveness. *Brain imaging and behavior*, *18*(3), 588–597. https://doi.org/10.1007/s11682-024-00856-z
3. Ricciardi, E., Rota, G., Sani, L., Gentili, C., Gaglianese, A., Guazzelli, M., & Pietrini, P. (2013). How the brain heals emotional wounds: the functional neuroanatomy of forgiveness. *Frontiers in human neuroscience*, *7*, 839. https://doi.org/10.3389/fnhum.2013.00839
4. Schuttenberg, E. M., Sneider, J. T., Rosmarin, D. H., Cohen-Gilbert, J. E., Oot, E. N., Seraikas, A. M., Stein, E. R., Maksimovskiy, A. L., Harris, S. K., & Silveri, M. M. (2022). Forgiveness Mediates the Relationship Between Middle Frontal Gyrus Volume and Clinical Symptoms in Adolescents. *Frontiers in human neuroscience*, *16*, 782893. https://doi.org/10.3389/fnhum.2022.782893

5. Akhtar, S., & Barlow, J. (2018). Forgiveness Therapy for the Promotion of Mental Well-Being: A Systematic Review and Meta-Analysis. *Trauma, violence & abuse*, *19*(1), 107–122. https://doi.org/10.1177/1524838016637079
6. Rasmussen, K. R., Stackhouse, M., Boon, S. D., Comstock, K., & Ross, R. (2019). Meta-analytic connections between forgiveness and health: the moderating effects of forgiveness-related distinctions. *Psychology & health*, *34*(5), 515–534. https://doi.org/10.1080/08870446.2018.1545906
7. Toussaint, L. L., Shields, G. S., & Slavich, G. M. (2016). Forgiveness, Stress, and Health: a 5-Week Dynamic Parallel Process Study. *Annals of behavioral medicine : a publication of the Society of Behavioral Medicine*, *50*(5), 727–735. https://doi.org/10.1007/s12160-016-9796-6
8. Toussaint, L., Shields, G. S., Dorn, G., & Slavich, G. M. (2016). Effects of lifetime stress exposure on mental and physical health in young adulthood: How stress degrades and forgiveness protects health. *Journal of health psychology*, *21*(6), 1004–1014. https://doi.org/10.1177/1359105314544132
9. Rasmussen, K. R., Stackhouse, M., Boon, S. D., Comstock, K., & Ross, R. (2019). Meta-analytic connections between forgiveness and health: the moderating effects of forgiveness-related distinctions. *Psychology & health*, *34*(5), 515–534. https://doi.org/10.1080/08870446.2018.1545906
10. Mullen, L. M., Bistany, B. R., Kim, J. J., Joseph, R. A., Akers, S. W., Harvey, J. R., & Houghton, A. (2023). Facilitation of Forgiveness: Impact on Health and Well-being. *Holistic nursing practice*, *37*(1), 15–23. https://doi.org/10.1097/HNP.0000000000000559
11. Waltman, M. A., Russell, D. C., Coyle, C. T., Enright, R. D., Holter, A. C., & M Swoboda, C. (2009). The effects of a forgiveness intervention on patients with coronary artery disease. *Psychology & health*, *24*(1), 11–27. https://doi.org/10.1080/08870440903126371
12. Lee, Y. R., & Enright, R. D. (2014). A Forgiveness Intervention for Women With Fibromyalgia Who Were Abused in Childhood: A Pilot Study. *Spirituality in clinical practice (Washington, D.C.)*, *1*(3), 203–217. https://doi.org/10.1037/scp0000025
13. Yazla, E., Karadere, M. E., Küçükler, F. K., Karşıdağ, Ç., İnanç, L., Kankoç, E., Dönertaş, M., & Demir, E. (2018). The Effect of Religious Belief and Forgiveness on Coping with Diabetes. *Journal of religion and health*, *57*(3), 1010–1019. https://doi.org/10.1007/s10943-017-0504-z
14. Lee, Y. R., & Enright, R. D. (2019). A meta-analysis of the association between forgiveness of others and physical health. *Psychology & health*, *34*(5), 626–643. https://doi.org/10.1080/08870446.2018.1554185
15. Elliott B. A. (2011). Forgiveness therapy: a clinical intervention for chronic disease. *Journal of religion and health*, *50*(2), 240–247. https://doi.org/10.1007/s10943-010-9336-9
16. Toussaint, L., Worthington, E. L., Jr, Van Tongeren, D. R., Hook, J., Berry, J. W., Shivy, V. A., Miller, A. J., & Davis, D. E. (2018). Forgiveness Working: Forgiveness, Health, and Productivity in the Workplace. *American journal of health promotion : AJHP*, *32*(1), 59–67. https://doi.org/10.1177/0890117116662312
17. Cao, W., van der Wal, R. C., & Taris, T. W. (2021). The Benefits of Forgiveness at Work: A Longitudinal Investigation of the Time-Lagged Relations Between Forgiveness and Work Outcomes. *Frontiers in psychology*, *12*, 710984. https://doi.org/10.3389/fpsyg.2021.710984
18. Crandall, A., Cheung, A., Miller, J. R., Glade, R., & Novilla, L. K. (2019). Dispositional forgiveness and stress as primary correlates of executive functioning in adults. *Health psychology open*, *6*(1), 2055102919848572. https://doi.org/10.1177/2055102919848572

36. The Five Steps
1. Schrøder, K., la Cour, K., Jørgensen, J. S., Lamont, R. F., & Hvidt, N. C. (2017). Guilt without fault: A qualitative study into the ethics of forgiveness after traumatic childbirth. *Social science & medicine (1982)*, *176*, 14–20. https://doi.org/10.1016/j.socscimed.2017.01.017
2. Griffin, B. J., Norman, S. B., Weber, M. C., Hinkson, K. D., Jr, Jendro, A. M., Pyne, J. M., Worthington, E. L., Jr, & Maguen, S. (2024). Properties of the modified self-forgiveness dual-process scale in populations at risk for moral injury. *Stress and health : journal of the International Society for the Investigation of Stress*, e3413. Advance online publication. https://doi.org/10.1002/smi.3413

3. Gabriels, J. B., & Strelan, P. (2018). For whom we forgive matters: relationship focus magnifies, but self-focus buffers against the negative effects of forgiving an exploitative partner. *The British journal of social psychology*, *57*(1), 154–173. https://doi.org/10.1111/bjso.12230

4. Berg, S. J., Zaso, M. J., Biehler, K. M., & Read, J. P. (2024). Self-Compassion and Self-Forgiveness in Alcohol Risk, Treatment and Recovery: A Systematic Review. *Clinical psychology & psychotherapy*, *31*(3), e2987. https://doi.org/10.1002/cpp.2987

5. Wilson, T., Milosevic, A., Carroll, M., Hart, K., & Hibbard, S. (2008). Physical health status in relation to self-forgiveness and other-forgiveness in healthy college students. *Journal of health psychology*, *13*(6), 798–803. https://doi.org/10.1177/1359105308093863

6. Skolnick, V. G., Lynch, B. A., Smith, L., Romanowicz, M., Blain, G., & Toussaint, L. (2023). The Association Between Parent and Child ACEs is Buffered by Forgiveness of Others and Self-Forgiveness. *Journal of child & adolescent trauma*, *16*(4), 1–9. Advance online publication. https://doi.org/10.1007/s40653-023-00552-y

7. Kaye-Tzadok, A., & Davidson-Arad, B. (2017). The Contribution of Cognitive Strategies to the Resilience of Women Survivors of Childhood Sexual Abuse and Non-Abused Women. *Violence against women*, *23*(8), 993–1015. https://doi.org/10.1177/1077801216652506

8. Long, K. N. G., Chen, Y., Potts, M., Hanson, J., & VanderWeele, T. J. (2020). Spiritually Motivated Self-Forgiveness and Divine Forgiveness, and Subsequent Health and Well-Being Among Middle-Aged Female Nurses: An Outcome-Wide Longitudinal Approach. *Frontiers in psychology*, *11*, 1337. https://doi.org/10.3389/fpsyg.2020.01337

9. Levi-Belz, Y., Dichter, N., & Zerach, G. (2022). Moral Injury and Suicide Ideation Among Israeli Combat Veterans: The Contribution of Self-Forgiveness and Perceived Social Support. *Journal of interpersonal violence*, *37*(1-2), NP1031–NP1057. https://doi.org/10.1177/0886260520920865

10. Levi-Belz, Y., & Gilo, T. (2020). Emotional Distress Among Suicide Survivors: The Moderating Role of Self-Forgiveness. *Frontiers in psychiatry*, *11*, 341. https://doi.org/10.3389/fpsyt.2020.00341

11. Cleare, S., Gumley, A., & O'Connor, R. C. (2019). Self-compassion, self-forgiveness, suicidal ideation, and self-harm: A systematic review. *Clinical psychology & psychotherapy*, *26*(5), 511–530. https://doi.org/10.1002/cpp.2372

12. Westers, N. J., Rehfuss, M., Olson, L., & Biron, D. (2012). The role of forgiveness in adolescents who engage in nonsuicidal self-injury. *The Journal of nervous and mental disease*, *200*(6), 535–541. https://doi.org/10.1097/NMD.0b013e318257c837

13. Osei-Tutu, A., Cowden, R. G., Kwakye-Nuako, C. O., Gadze, J., Oppong, S., & Worthington, E. L., Jr (2021). Self-Forgiveness Among Incarcerated Individuals in Ghana: Relations With Shame- and Guilt-Proneness. *International journal of offender therapy and comparative criminology*, *65*(5), 558–570. https://doi.org/10.1177/0306624X20914496

14. McGaffin, B. J., Lyons, G. C., & Deane, F. P. (2013). Self-forgiveness, shame, and guilt in recovery from drug and alcohol problems. *Substance abuse*, *34*(4), 396–404. https://doi.org/10.1080/08897077.2013.781564

15. Vallejo, M. A., Vallejo-Slocker, L., Rivera, J., Offenbächer, M., Dezutter, J., & Toussaint, L. (2020). Self-forgiveness in fibromyalgia patients and its relationship with acceptance, catastrophising and coping. *Clinical and experimental rheumatology*, *38 Suppl 123*(1), 79–85.

16. Toussaint, L., Gall, A. J., Cheadle, A., & Williams, D. R. (2020). Editor choice: Let it rest: Sleep and health as positive correlates of forgiveness of others and self-forgiveness. *Psychology & health*, *35*(3), 302–317. https://doi.org/10.1080/08870446.2019.1644335

17. Nolen-Hoeksema, S., Wisco, B. E., & Lyubomirsky, S. (2008). Rethinking Rumination. *Perspectives on Psychological Science*, *3*(5), 400-424. https://doi.org/10.1111/j.1745-6924.2008.00088.x

18. Toussaint, L., Barry, M., Angus, D., Bornfriend, L., & Markman, M. (2017). Self-forgiveness is associated with reduced psychological distress in cancer patients and unmatched caregivers: Hope and self-blame as mediating mechanisms. *Journal of psychosocial oncology*, *35*(5), 544–560. https://doi.org/10.1080/07347332.2017.1309615

19. Toussaint, L. L., Shields, G. S., Green, E., Kennedy, K., Travers, S., & Slavich, G. M. (2018). Hostility, forgiveness, and cognitive impairment over 10 years in a national sample of American

adults. *Health psychology : official journal of the Division of Health Psychology, American Psychological Association, 37*(12), 1102–1106.
20. Rahmati, A., & Poormirzaei, M. (2018). Predicting Nurses' Psychological Safety Based on the Forgiveness Skill. *Iranian journal of nursing and midwifery research, 23*(1), 40–44. https://doi.org/10.4103/ijnmr.IJNMR_240_16
21. Maynard, P. G., van Kessel, K., & Feather, J. S. (2023). Self-forgiveness, self-compassion and psychological health: A qualitative exploration of change during compassion focused therapy groups. *Psychology and psychotherapy, 96*(2), 265–280. https://doi.org/10.1111/papt.12435
22. Svalina, S. S., & Webb, J. R. (2012). Forgiveness and health among people in outpatient physical therapy. *Disability and rehabilitation, 34*(5), 383–392. https://doi.org/10.3109/09638288.2011.607216
23. Cornish, M.A. and Wade, N.G. (2015), A Therapeutic Model of Self-Forgiveness With Intervention Strategies for Counselors. Journal of Counseling & Development, 93: 96-104. https://doi.org/10.1002/j.1556-6676.2015.00185.x
24. Krause N. (2015). Assessing the relationships among race, religion, humility, and self-forgiveness: A longitudinal investigation. *Advances in life course research, 24*, 66–74. https://doi.org/10.1016/j.alcr.2015.02.003
25. Woodyatt, L., Wenzel, M., & Ferber, M. (2017). Two pathways to self-forgiveness: A hedonic path via self-compassion and a eudaimonic path via the reaffirmation of violated values. *The British journal of social psychology, 56*(3), 515–536. https://doi.org/10.1111/bjso.12194
26. Zhang, J. W., Chen, S., & Tomova Shakur, T. K. (2020). From Me to You: Self-Compassion Predicts Acceptance of Own and Others' Imperfections. *Personality and Social Psychology Bulletin, 46*(2), 228-242. https://doi.org/10.1177/0146167219853846
27. Marcinechová, D., Záhorcová, L., & Lohazerová, K. (2023). Self-forgiveness, Guilt, Shame, and Parental Stress among Parents of Children with Autism Spectrum Disorder. *Current psychology (New Brunswick, N.J.)*, 1–16. Advance online publication. https://doi.org/10.1007/s12144-023-04476-6
28. Schumacher, L. M., Arigo, D., & Thomas, C. (2017). Understanding physical activity lapses among women: responses to lapses and the potential buffering effect of social support. *Journal of behavioral medicine, 40*(5), 740–749. https://doi.org/10.1007/s10865-017-9846-y
29. Wohl, M. J., & Thompson, A. (2011). A dark side to self-forgiveness: forgiving the self and its association with chronic unhealthy behaviour. *The British journal of social psychology, 50*(Pt 2), 354–364. https://doi.org/10.1111/j.2044-8309.2010.02010.x
30. Squires, E. C., Sztainert, T., Gillen, N. R., Caouette, J., & Wohl, M. J. (2012). The problem with self-forgiveness: forgiving the self deters readiness to change among gamblers. *Journal of gambling studies, 28*(3), 337–350. https://doi.org/10.1007/s10899-011-9272-y
31. Vitz, P. C., & Meade, J. M. (2011). Self-forgiveness in psychology and psychotherapy: a critique. *Journal of religion and health, 50*(2), 248–263. https://doi.org/10.1007/s10943-010-9343-x

Appendix A: Loneliness Basics
1. Cacioppo, J. T., Cacioppo, S., & Boomsma, D. I. (2014). Evolutionary mechanisms for loneliness. *Cognition & emotion, 28*(1), 3–21. https://doi.org/10.1080/02699931.2013.837379
2. Baumeister, R. F., & Leary, M. R. (1995). The need to belong: desire for interpersonal attachments as a fundamental human motivation. *Psychological bulletin, 117*(3), 497–529.
3. Peplau LA, Perlman D. Perspectives on loneliness. In: Peplau LA, Perlman D, editors. *Loneliness: A sourcebook of current theory, research and therapy*. New York: Wiley; 1982. pp. 1–8.
4. Cacioppo, J. T., Cacioppo, S., Capitanio, J. P., & Cole, S. W. (2015). The neuroendocrinology of social isolation. *Annual review of psychology, 66*, 733–767. https://doi.org/10.1146/annurev-psych-010814-015240
5. Cacioppo, S., Grippo, A. J., London, S., Goossens, L., & Cacioppo, J. T. (2015). Loneliness: clinical import and interventions. *Perspectives on psychological science : a journal of the Association for Psychological Science, 10*(2), 238–249. https://doi.org/10.1177/1745691615570616

6. Buecker, S., Mund, M., Chwastek, S., Sostmann, M., & Luhmann, M. (2021). Is loneliness in emerging adults increasing over time? A preregistered cross-temporal meta-analysis and systematic review. *Psychological bulletin, 147*(8), 787–805. https://doi.org/10.1037/bul0000332
7. https://www.shrm.org/topics-tools/news/all-things-work/lonely-work (Accessed 7/25/2024)
8. https://blog.perceptyx.com/new-perceptyx-research-shines-a-light-on-loneliness-in-the-workplace (Accessed 07/24/2024)
9. Layden, E. A., Cacioppo, J. T., & Cacioppo, S. (2018). Loneliness predicts a preference for larger interpersonal distance within intimate space. *PloS one, 13*(9), e0203491. https://doi.org/10.1371/journal.pone.0203491
10. Nicolaisen, M., Pripp, A. H., & Thorsen, K. (2023). Why Not Lonely? A Longitudinal Study of Factors Related to Loneliness and Non-Loneliness in Different Age Groups Among People in the Second Part of Life. *International journal of aging & human development, 97*(2), 157–187. https://doi.org/10.1177/00914150221112292
11. Islam, M. K., & Gilmour, H. (2023). Immigrant status and loneliness among older Canadians. *Health reports, 34*(7), 3–18. https://doi.org/10.25318/82-003-x202300700001-eng
12. McKenna-Plumley, P. E., Turner, R. N., Yang, K., & Groarke, J. M. (2023). Experiences of Loneliness Across the Lifespan: A Systematic Review and Thematic Synthesis of Qualitative Studies. *International journal of qualitative studies on health and well-being, 18*(1), 2223868. https://doi.org/10.1080/17482631.2023.2223868

Appendix B: How Loneliness Perpetuates Itself

1. Masi, C. M., Chen, H. Y., Hawkley, L. C., & Cacioppo, J. T. (2011). A meta-analysis of interventions to reduce loneliness. *Personality and social psychology review : an official journal of the Society for Personality and Social Psychology, Inc, 15*(3), 219–266. https://doi.org/10.1177/1088868310377394
2. Cacioppo, S., Grippo, A. J., London, S., Goossens, L., & Cacioppo, J. T. (2015). Loneliness: clinical import and interventions. *Perspectives on psychological science : a journal of the Association for Psychological Science, 10*(2), 238–249. https://doi.org/10.1177/1745691615570616
3. Bell, V., Velthorst, E., Almansa, J., Myin-Germeys, I., Shergill, S., & Fett, A. K. (2023). Do loneliness and social exclusion breed paranoia? An experience sampling investigation across the psychosis continuum. *Schizophrenia research. Cognition, 33*, 100282. https://doi.org/10.1016/j.scog.2023.100282
4. Bangee M, Harris RA, Bridges N, Rotenberg KJ, Qualter P. Loneliness and attention to social threat in young adults: findings from an eye tracker study. *Personal Individ Differ*. 2014;63:16–23.
5. Cacioppo, J. T., & Cacioppo, S. (2014). Social Relationships and Health: The Toxic Effects of Perceived Social Isolation. *Social and personality psychology compass, 8*(2), 58–72. https://doi.org/10.1111/spc3.12087
6. Cacioppo, S., Bangee, M., Balogh, S., Cardenas-Iniguez, C., Qualter, P., & Cacioppo, J. T. (2016). Loneliness and implicit attention to social threat: A high-performance electrical neuroimaging study. *Cognitive neuroscience, 7*(1-4), 138–159. https://doi.org/10.1080/17588928.2015.1070136
7. Cacioppo, J. T., Cacioppo, S., Capitanio, J. P., & Cole, S. W. (2015). The neuroendocrinology of social isolation. *Annual review of psychology, 66*, 733–767. https://doi.org/10.1146/annurev-psych-010814-015240
8. Layden, E. A., Cacioppo, J. T., & Cacioppo, S. (2018). Loneliness predicts a preference for larger interpersonal distance within intimate space. *PloS one, 13*(9), e0203491. https://doi.org/10.1371/journal.pone.0203491
9. Cacioppo, J. T., & Cacioppo, S. (2014). Social Relationships and Health: The Toxic Effects of Perceived Social Isolation. *Social and personality psychology compass, 8*(2), 58–72. https://doi.org/10.1111/spc3.12087
10. Cacioppo, J. T., & Cacioppo, S. (2014). Social Relationships and Health: The Toxic Effects of Perceived Social Isolation. *Social and personality psychology compass, 8*(2), 58–72. https://doi.org/10.1111/spc3.12087

11. Finley, A. J., & Schaefer, S. M. (2022). Affective Neuroscience of Loneliness: Potential Mechanisms underlying the Association between Perceived Social Isolation, Health, and Well-Being. *Journal of psychiatry and brain science, 7*(6), e220011. https://doi.org/10.20900/jpbs.20220011
12. Nowland, R., Robinson, S. J., Bradley, B. F., Summers, V., & Qualter, P. (2018). Loneliness, HPA stress reactivity and social threat sensitivity: Analyzing naturalistic social challenges. *Scandinavian Journal of Psychology, 59*(5), 540–546. https://doi.org/10.1111/sjop.12461
13. Gardner, W. L., Pickett, C. L., Jefferis, V., & Knowles, M. (2005). On the Outside Looking In: Loneliness and Social Monitoring. *Personality and Social Psychology Bulletin, 31*(11), 1549-1560. https://doi.org/10.1177/0146167205277208
14. Barreto, M., van Breen, J., Victor, C., Hammond, C., Eccles, A., Richins, M. T., & Qualter, P. (2022). Exploring the nature and variation of the stigma associated with loneliness. *Journal of social and personal relationships, 39*(9), 2658–2679. https://doi.org/10.1177/02654075221087190
Kerr NA, Stanley TB. Revisiting the social stigma of loneliness. *Pers Indiv Differ.* 2021;171:110482
15. Barreto M, van Breen J, Victor C, Hammond C, Eccles A, Richins MT, et al. Exploring the nature and variation of the stigma associated with loneliness. *J Soc Pers Relat.* 2022;39:2658–79.
16. Wang W, Zhou K, Yu Z, Li J. The cost of Impression Management to Life satisfaction: sense of control and loneliness as mediators. *Psychol Res Behav Manag.* 2020;13:407–17.
17. Rotenberg KJ, Bartley JL, Toivonen D. Children's stigmatization of chronic loneliness. *J Social Behav Personality.* 1997;12:577.
18. Lau S, Gruen GE. The Social Stigma of loneliness: Effect of Target Person's and Perceiver's sex. *Pers Soc Psychol Bull.* 1992;18:182–9.

Appendix C: Loneliness and Connection with Self

1. Thoresen, S., Aakvaag, H. F., Strøm, I. F., Wentzel-Larsen, T., & Birkeland, M. S. (2018). Loneliness as a mediator of the relationship between shame and health problems in young people exposed to childhood violence. *Social science & medicine (1982), 211*, 183–189. https://doi.org/10.1016/j.socscimed.2018.06.002
2. Cohen-Mansfield, J., Hazan, H., Lerman, Y., & Shalom, V. (2016). Correlates and predictors of loneliness in older-adults: a review of quantitative results informed by qualitative insights. *International psychogeriatrics, 28*(4), 557–576. https://doi.org/10.1017/S1041610215001532
3. Pedroso-Chaparro, M. D. S., Cabrera, I., Vara-García, C., Márquez-González, M., & Losada-Baltar, A. (2023). Physical limitations and loneliness: The role of guilt related to self-perception as a burden. *Journal of the American Geriatrics Society, 71*(3), 903–908. https://doi.org/10.1111/jgs.18149
4. Fan, W., Ma, K. K., Yang, C. X., & Guo, Y. L. (2023). The mediating effect of stigma between self-perceived burden and loneliness in stroke patients. *Frontiers in psychiatry, 14*, 1219805. https://doi.org/10.3389/fpsyt.2023.1219805
5. Salway, S., Such, E., Preston, L., Booth, A., Zubair, M., Victor, C., & Raghavan, R. (2020). *Reducing loneliness among migrant and ethnic minority people: a participatory evidence synthesis.* NIHR Journals Library.
6. Ingram, I., Kelly, P. J., Deane, F. P., Baker, A. L., & Dingle, G. A. (2020). Perceptions of loneliness among people accessing treatment for substance use disorders. *Drug and alcohol review, 39*(5), 484–494. https://doi.org/10.1111/dar.13120
7. Qualter, P., Brown, S. L., Rotenberg, K. J., Vanhalst, J., Harris, R. A., Goossens, L., Bangee, M., & Munn, P. (2013). Trajectories of loneliness during childhood and adolescence: predictors and health outcomes. *Journal of adolescence, 36*(6), 1283–1293. https://doi.org/10.1016/j.adolescence.2013.01.005
8. Dibb, B., & Foster, M. (2021). Loneliness and Facebook use: the role of social comparison and rumination. *Heliyon, 7*(1), e05999. https://doi.org/10.1016/j.heliyon.2021.e05999
9. Yang C. C. (2016). Instagram Use, Loneliness, and Social Comparison Orientation: Interact and Browse on Social Media, But Don't Compare. *Cyberpsychology, behavior and social networking, 19*(12), 703–708. https://doi.org/10.1089/cyber.2016.0201

10. Wollast, R., Preece, D. A., Schmitz, M., Bigot, A., Gross, J. J., & Luminet, O. (2024). The role of self-compassion in loneliness during the COVID-19 pandemic: a group-based trajectory modelling approach. *Cognition & emotion*, *38*(1), 103–119. https://doi.org/10.1080/02699931.2023.2270201

11. Patapoff, M. A., Jester, D. J., Daly, R. E., Mausbach, B. T., Depp, C. A., & Glorioso, D. K. (2024). Remotely-administered resilience and self-compassion intervention targeting loneliness and stress in older adults: a single-case experimental design. *Aging & mental health*, *28*(2), 369–376. https://doi.org/10.1080/13607863.2023.2262411

12. Gao, P., Mosazadeh, H., & Nazari, N. (2023). The Buffering Role of Self-compassion in the Association Between Loneliness with Depressive Symptoms: A Cross-Sectional Survey Study Among Older Adults Living in Residential Care Homes During COVID-19. *International journal of mental health and addiction*, 1–21. Advance online publication. https://doi.org/10.1007/s11469-023-01014-0

13. Borawski, D., & Nowak, A. (2022). As long as you are self-compassionate, you will never walk alone. The interplay between self-compassion and rejection sensitivity in predicting loneliness. *International journal of psychology : Journal international de psychologie*, *57*(5), 621–628. https://doi.org/10.1002/ijop.12850

14. Lyon, Taylor A., "Self-Compassion as a Predictor of Loneliness: The Relationship Between Self-Evaluation Processes and Perceptions of Social Connection" (2015). Selected Honors Theses. Paper 37. https://firescholars.seu.edu/cgi/viewcontent.cgi?article=1038&context=honors (Accessed 7/25/2024)

15. Andel, S. A., Shen, W., & Arvan, M. L. (2021). Depending on your own kindness: The moderating role of self-compassion on the within-person consequences of work loneliness during the COVID-19 pandemic. *Journal of occupational health psychology*, *26*(4), 276–290. https://doi.org/10.1037/ocp0000271

16. Wang, S., Tang, Q., Lv, Y., Tao, Y., Liu, X., Zhang, L., & Liu, G. (2023). The Temporal Relationship between Depressive Symptoms and Loneliness: The Moderating Role of Self-Compassion. *Behavioral sciences (Basel, Switzerland)*, *13*(6), 472. https://doi.org/10.3390/bs13060472

17. Li, S., Zhang, X., Luo, C., Chen, M., Xie, X., Gong, F., Lv, F., Xu, J., Han, J., Fu, L., & Sun, Y. (2021). The mediating role of self-acceptance in the relationship between loneliness and subjective well-being among the elderly in nursing home: A cross-sectional study. *Medicine*, *100*(40), e27364. https://doi.org/10.1097/MD.0000000000027364

18. Kong, L., Gao, Z., Xu, N., Shao, S., Ma, H., He, Q., Zhang, D., Xu, H., & Qu, H. (2021). The relation between self-stigma and loneliness in visually impaired college students: Self-acceptance as mediator. *Disability and health journal*, *14*(2), 101054. https://doi.org/10.1016/j.dhjo.2020.101054

19. Rosenthal, S., Schlussel, Y., Yaden, M. B., DeSantis, J., Trayes, K., Pohl, C., & Hojat, M. (2021). Persistent Impostor Phenomenon Is Associated With Distress in Medical Students. *Family medicine*, *53*(2), 118–122. https://doi.org/10.22454/FamMed.2021.799997

20. Borawski, D., Sojda, M., Rychlewska, K., & Wajs, T. (2022). Attached but Lonely: Emotional Intelligence as a Mediator and Moderator between Attachment Styles and Loneliness. *International journal of environmental research and public health*, *19*(22), 14831. https://doi.org/10.3390/ijerph192214831

Appendix D: What Works?

1. Morrish, N., Choudhury, S., & Medina-Lara, A. (2023). What works in interventions targeting loneliness: a systematic review of intervention characteristics. *BMC public health*, *23*(1), 2214. https://doi.org/10.1186/s12889-023-17097-2

2. Masi, C. M., Chen, H. Y., Hawkley, L. C., & Cacioppo, J. T. (2011). A meta-analysis of interventions to reduce loneliness. *Personality and social psychology review : an official journal of the Society for Personality and Social Psychology, Inc*, *15*(3), 219–266. https://doi.org/10.1177/1088868310377394

3. Yu, D. S., Li, P. W., Lin, R. S., Kee, F., Chiu, A., & Wu, W. (2023). Effects of non-pharmacological interventions on loneliness among community-dwelling older adults: A systematic review, network meta-analysis, and meta-regression. *International journal of nursing studies*, *144*, 104524. https://doi.org/10.1016/j.ijnurstu.2023.104524

4. Hickin, N., Käll, A., Shafran, R., Sutcliffe, S., Manzotti, G., & Langan, D. (2021). The effectiveness of psychological interventions for loneliness: A systematic review and meta-analysis. *Clinical psychology review, 88*, 102066. https://doi.org/10.1016/j.cpr.2021.102066

5. Hards, E., Loades, M. E., Higson-Sweeney, N., Shafran, R., Serafimova, T., Brigden, A., Reynolds, S., Crawley, E., Chatburn, E., Linney, C., McManus, M., & Borwick, C. (2022). Loneliness and mental health in children and adolescents with pre-existing mental health problems: A rapid systematic review. *The British journal of clinical psychology, 61*(2), 313–334. https://doi.org/10.1111/bjc.12331

6. Li, M., Rao, W., Su, Y., Sul, Y., Caron, G., D'Arcy, C., Fleury, M. J., & Meng, X. (2023). Psychological interventions for loneliness and social isolation among older adults during medical pandemics: a systematic review and meta-analysis. *Age and ageing, 52*(6), afad076. https://doi.org/10.1093/ageing/afad076

7. Yu, D. S., Li, P. W., Lin, R. S., Kee, F., Chiu, A., & Wu, W. (2023). Effects of non-pharmacological interventions on loneliness among community-dwelling older adults: A systematic review, network meta-analysis, and meta-regression. *International journal of nursing studies, 144*, 104524. https://doi.org/10.1016/j.ijnurstu.2023.104524

8. Li, J., Zhou, X., & Wang, Q. (2023). Interventions to reduce loneliness among Chinese older adults: A network meta-analysis of randomized controlled trials and quasi-experimental studies. *Applied psychology. Health and well-being, 15*(1), 238–258. https://doi.org/10.1111/aphw.12375

9. Ellard, O. B., Dennison, C., & Tuomainen, H. (2023). Review: Interventions addressing loneliness amongst university students: a systematic review. *Child and adolescent mental health, 28*(4), 512–523. https://doi.org/10.1111/camh.12614

10. Cacioppo, S., Grippo, A. J., London, S., Goossens, L., & Cacioppo, J. T. (2015). Loneliness: clinical import and interventions. *Perspectives on psychological science : a journal of the Association for Psychological Science, 10*(2), 238–249. https://doi.org/10.1177/1745691615570616

11. Sha, S., Loveys, K., Qualter, P., Shi, H., Krpan, D., & Galizzi, M. (2024). Efficacy of relational agents for loneliness across age groups: a systematic review and meta-analysis. *BMC public health, 24*(1), 1802. https://doi.org/10.1186/s12889-024-19153-x

12. Yen, H. Y., Huang, C. W., Chiu, H. L., & Jin, G. (2024). The Effect of Social Robots on Depression and Loneliness for Older Residents in Long-Term Care Facilities: A Meta-Analysis of Randomized Controlled Trials. *Journal of the American Medical Directors Association, 25*(6), 104979. https://doi.org/10.1016/j.jamda.2024.02.017

13. Reference

14. Marziali, R. A., Franceschetti, C., Dinculescu, A., Nistorescu, A., Kristály, D. M., Moşoi, A. A., Broekx, R., Marin, M., Vizitiu, C., Moraru, S. A., Rossi, L., & Di Rosa, M. (2024). Reducing Loneliness and Social Isolation of Older Adults Through Voice Assistants: Literature Review and Bibliometric Analysis. *Journal of medical Internet research, 26*, e50534. https://doi.org/10.2196/50534

15. Shah, S. G. S., Nogueras, D., van Woerden, H. C., & Kiparoglou, V. (2021). Evaluation of the Effectiveness of Digital Technology Interventions to Reduce Loneliness in Older Adults: Systematic Review and Meta-analysis. *Journal of medical Internet research, 23*(6), e24712. https://doi.org/10.2196/24712

16. Jin, W., Liu, Y., Yuan, S., Bai, R., Li, X., & Bai, Z. (2021). The Effectiveness of Technology-Based Interventions for Reducing Loneliness in Older Adults: A Systematic Review and Meta-Analysis of Randomized Controlled Trials. *Frontiers in psychology, 12*, 711030. https://doi.org/10.3389/fpsyg.2021.711030

17. Noone, C., McSharry, J., Smalle, M., Burns, A., Dwan, K., Devane, D., & Morrissey, E. C. (2020). Video calls for reducing social isolation and loneliness in older people: a rapid review. *The Cochrane database of systematic reviews, 5*(5), CD013632. https://doi.org/10.1002/14651858.CD013632

18. Döring, N., Conde, M., Brandenburg, K., Broll, W., Gross, H. M., Werner, S., & Raake, A. (2022). Can Communication Technologies Reduce Loneliness and Social Isolation in Older People? A Scoping Review of Reviews. *International journal of environmental research and public health, 19*(18), 11310. https://doi.org/10.3390/ijerph191811310

19. Shekelle, P. G., Miake-Lye, I. M., Begashaw, M. M., Booth, M. S., Myers, B., Lowery, N., & Shrank, W. H. (2024). Interventions to Reduce Loneliness in Community-Living Older Adults: a

Systematic Review and Meta-analysis. *Journal of general internal medicine, 39*(6), 1015–1028. https://doi.org/10.1007/s11606-023-08517-5

20. Fu, Z., Yan, M., & Meng, C. (2022). The effectiveness of remote delivered intervention for loneliness reduction in older adults: A systematic review and meta-analysis. *Frontiers in psychology, 13*, 935544. https://doi.org/10.3389/fpsyg.2022.935544

21. Nowland, R., Necka, E. A., & Cacioppo, J. T. (2018). Loneliness and Social Internet Use: Pathways to Reconnection in a Digital World?. *Perspectives on psychological science : a journal of the Association for Psychological Science, 13*(1), 70–87. https://doi.org/10.1177/1745691617713052

22. Sun, P., Xing, L., Wu, J., & Kou, Y. (2023). Receiving feedback after posting status updates on social networking sites predicts lower loneliness: A mediated moderation model. *Applied psychology. Health and well-being, 15*(1), 97–114. https://doi.org/10.1111/aphw.12378

23. Bower, M., Kent, J., Patulny, R., Green, O., McGrath, L., Teesson, L., Jamalishahni, T., Sandison, H., & Rugel, E. (2023). The impact of the built environment on loneliness: A systematic review and narrative synthesis. *Health & place, 79*, 102962. https://doi.org/10.1016/j.healthplace.2022.102962

24. Astell-Burt, T., Hartig, T., Putra, I. G. N. E., Walsan, R., Dendup, T., & Feng, X. (2022). Green space and loneliness: A systematic review with theoretical and methodological guidance for future research. *The Science of the total environment, 847*, 157521. https://doi.org/10.1016/j.scitotenv.2022.157521

25. Astell-Burt, T., Hartig, T., Eckermann, S., Nieuwenhuijsen, M., McMunn, A., Frumkin, H., & Feng, X. (2022). More green, less lonely? A longitudinal cohort study. *International journal of epidemiology, 51*(1), 99–110. https://doi.org/10.1093/ije/dyab089

26. Hsueh, Y. C., Batchelor, R., Liebmann, M., Dhanani, A., Vaughan, L., Fett, A. K., Mann, F., & Pitman, A. (2022). A Systematic Review of Studies Describing the Effectiveness, Acceptability, and Potential Harms of Place-Based Interventions to Address Loneliness and Mental Health Problems. *International journal of environmental research and public health, 19*(8), 4766. https://doi.org/10.3390/ijerph19084766

27. Quan, N. G., Lohman, M. C., Resciniti, N. V., & Friedman, D. B. (2020). A systematic review of interventions for loneliness among older adults living in long-term care facilities. *Aging & mental health, 24*(12), 1945–1955. https://doi.org/10.1080/13607863.2019.1673311

28. Hoang, P., King, J. A., Moore, S., Moore, K., Reich, K., Sidhu, H., Tan, C. V., Whaley, C., & McMillan, J. (2022). Interventions Associated With Reduced Loneliness and Social Isolation in Older Adults: A Systematic Review and Meta-analysis. *JAMA network open, 5*(10), e2236676. https://doi.org/10.1001/jamanetworkopen.2022.36676

29. Kretzler, B., König, H. H., & Hajek, A. (2022). Pet ownership, loneliness, and social isolation: a systematic review. *Social psychiatry and psychiatric epidemiology, 57*(10), 1935–1957. https://doi.org/10.1007/s00127-022-02332-9

30. Delanoeije, J., & Verbruggen, M. (2024). Biophilia in the home-workplace: Integrating dog caregiving and outdoor access to explain teleworkers' daily physical activity, loneliness, and job performance. *Journal of occupational health psychology, 29*(3), 131–154. https://doi.org/10.1037/ocp0000378

31. Yu, J., Han, M., Miao, F., & Hua, D. (2023). Using mindfulness-based stress reduction to relieve loneliness, anxiety, and depression in cancer patients: A systematic review and meta-analysis. *Medicine, 102*(37), e34917. https://doi.org/10.1097/MD.0000000000034917

32. Itzchakov, G., Weinstein, N., Saluk, D., & Amar, M. (2023). Connection Heals Wounds: Feeling Listened to Reduces Speakers' Loneliness Following a Social Rejection Disclosure. *Personality & social psychology bulletin, 49*(8), 1273–1294. https://doi.org/10.1177/01461672221100369

33. Öztürk, F. Ö., Bayraktar, E. P., & Tezel, A. (2023). The effect of laughter yoga on loneliness, psychological resilience, and quality of life in older adults: A pilot randomized controlled trial. *Geriatric nursing (New York, N.Y.), 50*, 208–214. https://doi.org/10.1016/j.gerinurse.2023.01.009

34. Smith, M. L., Chen, E., Lau, C. A., Davis, D., Simmons, J. W., & Merianos, A. L. (2023). Effectiveness of chronic disease self-management education (CDSME) programs to reduce loneliness. *Chronic illness, 19*(3), 646–664. https://doi.org/10.1177/17423953221113604

35. Gray, N. L. T., & Roberts, S. C. (2023). An investigation of simulated and real touch on feelings of loneliness. *Scientific reports*, *13*(1), 10587. https://doi.org/10.1038/s41598-023-37467-5
36. Lanser, I., & Eisenberger, N. I. (2023). Prosocial behavior reliably reduces loneliness: An investigation across two studies. *Emotion (Washington, D.C.)*, *23*(6), 1781–1790. https://doi.org/10.1037/emo0001179
37. Chua, C. M. S., Chua, J. Y. X., & Shorey, S. (2024). Effectiveness of home-based interventions in improving loneliness and social connectedness among older adults: a systematic review and meta-analysis. *Aging & mental health*, *28*(1), 1–10. https://doi.org/10.1080/13607863.2023.2237919
38. Velloze, I. G., Jester, D. J., Jeste, D. V., & Mausbach, B. T. (2022). Interventions to reduce loneliness in caregivers: An integrative review of the literature. *Psychiatry research*, *311*, 114508. https://doi.org/10.1016/j.psychres.2022.114508
39. Lekhak, N., Bhatta, T. R., Kahana, E., & Snyder, J. S. (2023). The Primacy of Compassionate Love: Loneliness and Psychological Well-Being in Later Life. *Journal of gerontological nursing*, *49*(4), 12–20. https://doi.org/10.3928/00989134-20230309-03
40. Yu, D. S., Li, P. W., Lin, R. S., Kee, F., Chiu, A., & Wu, W. (2023). Effects of non-pharmacological interventions on loneliness among community-dwelling older adults: A systematic review, network meta-analysis, and meta-regression. *International journal of nursing studies*, *144*, 104524. https://doi.org/10.1016/j.ijnurstu.2023.104524
41. Pluim, C. F., Anzai, J. A. U., Martinez, J. E., Munera, D., Garza-Naveda, A. P., Vila-Castelar, C., Guzmán-Vélez, E., Ramirez-Gomez, L., Bustin, J., Serrano, C. M., Babulal, G. M., Okada de Oliveira, M., & Quiroz, Y. T. (2023). Associations Among Loneliness, Purpose in Life and Subjective Cognitive Decline in Ethnoracially Diverse Older Adults Living in the United States. *Journal of applied gerontology : the official journal of the Southern Gerontological Society*, *42*(3), 376–386. https://doi.org/10.1177/07334648221139479

Acknowledgements

I am grateful to the countless scientists, reporters, philosophers, and authors who have helped me learn the information I share in this book.

Several colleagues and friends who are actively involved in researching and building well-being and loneliness programs or help patients struggling with mental health issues have provided remarkable insights and quotes for the book. My special thanks to Arianna Huffington, Professor Lord Richard Layard, Professor Julianne Holt-Lunstad, Professor Fredric Luskin, Dr. Smriti Joshi, Daniel Schwartz, Dr. Jacinta Jimenez, Karen Cunningham, Payal Sahni Becher, Dr. Heather Farley, Dr. Jennifer Posa, Anu Jain, Chaplain Jim Hogg, Debbie Fuehrer, Reeva Misra, Dr. Gurmeet Narang, and Dr. Jonathan Fisher.

I have learned a lot from my collaborators at Mayo Clinic, New York Presbyterian Health System, Delta Airlines, Thrive Global, UC Berkeley, Atria Academy of Science and Medicine, Mikropis (Andrej Pantar), North Dakota Area Health Education Center, and InSciEd Out (Dr. Chris Pierret). I am grateful to all of them.

Daniel Schwartz, Gauri Sood, and Saara Chaudry provided a thoughtful and thorough review of the manuscript taking it several notches higher for which I am very appreciative.

I am eternally thankful to my many colleagues, friends, and extended family, my parents, Sahib and Shashi; my in-laws, Vinod and Kusum; my brothers, Kishore and Sundeep; my sisters, Sandhya, Rajni, Preeti, and Smita; my daughters, Gauri and Sia; my furry son Simba, and my wife, Richa, for showering me with love that sustains me every day.

I am indebted to every person helping build a kinder, happier, and more hopeful world for our planet's children. Thank you!

Amit

About The Author

―――❖❖❖―――

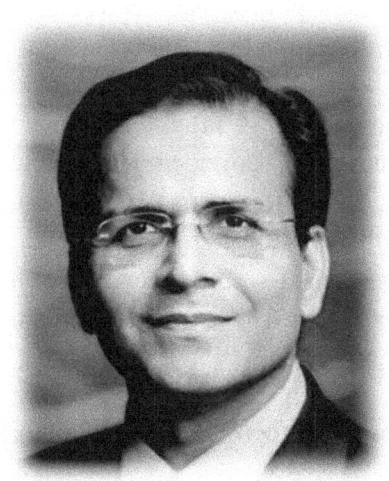

Dr. Amit Sood is married to his lovely wife of 31 years, Dr. Richa Sood. They have two daughters, Gauri (age 20) and Sia (age 14).

Dr. Sood is the Executive Director of the Global Center for Resiliency and Well-being and The GRIT Institute. He is internationally known for his work on stress management, resilience, well-being, mindfulness, and burnout.

He is a former Professor of Medicine at the Mayo Clinic, director of the Mayo Mind-Body Medicine Initiative, and enterprise chair of student life and wellness.

Dr. Sood completed his residency in internal medicine at the Albert Einstein School of Medicine, an integrative medicine fellowship at the University of Arizona, and earned a master's degree in clinical research from the Mayo Clinic College of Medicine. He has received several National Institutes of Health grants and foundation awards to test and implement integrative and mind-body approaches within medicine.

Dr. Sood's work has resulted in many resilience and well-being programs, including Transform, Resilient Option, Stress Management and Resiliency Training (SMART©), and Certified Resilience Trainer Course (CeRT). The programs have been adopted by several hospitals, health systems, and corporations as their resiliency and well-being platforms. SMART has been tested in over thirty five clinical trials and currently reaches approximately 250,000 participants each year with demonstrated efficacy for a broad demographic, including patients, caregivers, corporate executives, health care professionals, and students.

Dr. Sood has authored or co-authored over 80 peer-reviewed articles, editorials, book chapters, abstracts, and letters. He has also authored multiple books including *The Mayo Clinic Guide to Stress-Free Living*, *The Mayo Clinic Handbook for Happiness*, *Immerse: A 52-Week Course in Resilient Living*, *Mindfulness Redesigned for the Twenty-First Century*, *SMART with Dr. Sood*, *The Resilience Journal,* and *That Makes Sense.*

As an international expert in his field, Dr. Sood's work has been widely cited in the press, including *The Atlantic Monthly, USA Today, Wall Street Journal, New York Times, Forbes, NPR, Reuters Health, Time Magazine (online), Good Housekeeping, Parenting, Real Simple, Shape, US News, Huffington Post, AARP, The Globe and Mail, Fox News,* and *CBS News.* He is highly sought after as a speaker on resilience and stress management, having presented on some of the highest impact forums, including TEDx, Lake Nona, Forbes Under 30 Forum, Conference Board, Beckers, YPO, NPR, NAMI, NBGH, NASA, keynotes for Fortune 500 companies, universities, foundations, and others. Dr. Sood's videos, including the TEDx talk, *Happy Brain: How to Overcome Our Neural Predispositions to Suffering, A Very Happy Brain, NPR Presents, and CBS Sunday Morning with Jane Pauley,* have been seen by millions of viewers all over the world.

Dr. Sood received the 2010 Distinguished Service Award, the 2010 Innovator of the Year Award, the 2013 Outstanding Physician Scientist Award, and the 2016 Faculty of the Year Award from Mayo Clinic. He also was honored as the Robert Wood Johnson Health Care Pioneer in 2015. *The Intelligent Optimist* (formerly *Ode Magazine*) selected Dr. Sood as one among top 20 intelligent optimists helping the world to be a better place. In 2016, Dr. Sood was selected as the top impact maker in healthcare in Rochester, MN. Dr. Sood serves on the well-being advisory board for Everyday Health, scientific advisory board for Thrive Global, and is a fellow with the Atria Academy of Science and Medicine.

ADDITIONAL RESOURCES

Books:
SMART with Dr. Sood
The Resilience Journal
Immerse: A 52-Week Course in Resilient Living
Mindfulness Redesigned for the Twenty-First Century
Stronger: The Science and Art of Stress Resilience
Build Your Immune Resilience
That Makes Sense

Websites:
amitsood.com (Resilient Option Program)
resiliencetrainer.com (Certified Resilience Trainer Program)